The Complete Guide to
EYE CARE,
EYEGLASSES AND
CONTACT LENSES

DEDICATION

This book was possible because of the understanding and cooperation of our families. Though deprived of their full share of paternal attention while we spent many hours with the manuscript, they accepted the situation with only minimum grumbling. Our wives, Barbara and Phoebe, gave up innumerable weekends while we were immersed in authorship. Their encouragement, affection and willingness to be sounding boards for our ideas, helped us through many stalemates. Finally, a manuscript of this size requires a lot of typing time, much of which was cheerfully done (voluntarily) by Susan Zinn.

The
Complete Guide to
EYE CARE, EYEGLASSES and CONTACT LENSES

WALTER J. ZINN,
and
HERBERT SOLOMON, O.D., D.O.S., F.A.A.O.

Illustrated

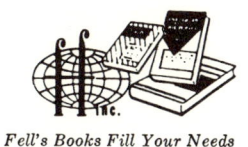

Fell's Books Fill Your Needs

FREDERICK FELL PUBLISHERS, INC.,
New York, New York

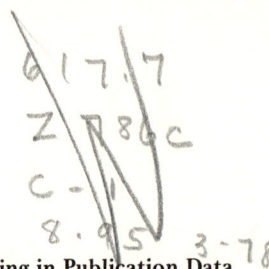

Library of Congress Cataloging in Publication Data

Zinn, Walter J.
  The complete guide to eye care, eyeglasses and contact lenses.

  1. Eye—Care and Care and hygiene. 2. Eye—Diseases and defects.
3. Ophthalmic lenses. I. Solomon, Herbert, joint author. II. Title.
[DNLM: 1. Ophthalmology—Popular works. 2. Optometry—Popular
works. WW80 Z78c]
RE51.Z56   617.7   77-8753
ISBN 0-8119-0281-1

Copyright © 1977, by Dr. Walter J. Zinn and Dr. Herbert Solomon

All rights reserved. No part of this work covered by the copyright herein may be reproduced or used in any form or by any means—graphic, electronic, or mechanical, including photocopying, recording, taping or information storage and retrieval systems—without permission of the publisher.

For information address:

Frederick Fell Publishers, Inc.
386 Park Avenue South
New York, New York 10016

Published simultaneously in Canada by:
Thomas Nelson & Sons, Limited
Don Mills, Ontario, Canada

MANUFACTURED IN THE UNITED STATES OF AMERICA

1 2 3 4 5 6 7 8 9 0

Designed by Michael Y. Polvere

CONTENTS

FOREWORD

PART I—YOUR VISUAL WORLD
Chapter 1—What's Your Vision All About?   1
Chapter 2—Do You See What You Are Looking At?   4
Chapter 3—The Eye   7
Chapter 4—Why Two Eyes?   14
Chapter 5—"I See," Said The Brain   18
Chapter 6—Visual Illusions   23
Chapter 7—Color Vision   30

PART II—HOW YOUR EYES SHOULD WORK AND WHAT CAN GO WRONG
Chapter 8—Normal Focusing And Eye Movements   35
Chapter 9—Common Sight Disorders And Corrections   39

PART III—THE EYE EXAMINATION
Chapter 10—How To Choose A Family Optometrist   47
Chapter 11—The "Drops" Myth   51
Chapter 12—The Vision Examination—What It Must Include   55
   A Complete Optometric Examination Chart   60
Chapter 13—Special Tests For Special Cases   61

PART IV—ALL ABOUT GLASSES AND CONTACT LENSES
Chapter 14—How Do Glasses Work?   67
Chapter 15—Getting Used To Your Glasses   71
Chapter 16—Bifocals And Multifocals   75
Chapter 17—Sunglasses And Tinted Lenses   81
   Selection Guide to Tinted-Glass Lenses   89
Chapter 18—Shatter-Resistant Glass or Plastic Lenses   91
Chapter 19—What Contact Lenses Are And How They Work   95

Chapter 20—Hard Lenses vs. Soft 101
                Hard vs. Soft Contact Lens Guide 105
Chapter 21—Guide To Successful Wear 107

PART V—CHILDREN'S VISION
Chapter 22—The Developing Visual System—How It Matures 119
Chapter 23—The Examination Of The Infant And Pre-Schooler 122
Chapter 24—Amblyopia—"Lazy Eye" 128
Chapter 25—Crossed Eyes 132
Chapter 26—Reading Problems Equal School Failures 136
Chapter 27—Bifocals For Children? 149

PART VI—VISION PROBLEMS OF THE AGED
Chapter 28—The Vision Of The Aging 155
Chapter 29—Cataracts, Cataract Surgery And How To Cope 159

PART VII—VISUAL THERAPY
Chapter 30—What It Is And When It's Indicated 167
Chapter 31—Control Of Nearsightedness 174

PART VIII—COMMON EYE DISEASES AND DISORDERS
Chapter 32—External Parts 185
                Lids 185
                Conjunctiva 186
                Cornea 187
                Sclera 188
Chapter 33—Internal Parts 189
                Iris 189
                Lens 190
                Vitreous 190
                Retina 190
                Optic Nerve 192
                Orbit 192
                Glaucoma 193

PART IX—THE PARTIALLY SIGHTED

Chapter 34—What It Is And Who Can Be Helped	197
Chapter 35—The Visually-Impaired Child	200
Chapter 36—Educational And Vocational Outlook	203
Chapter 37—Recent Sight Loss	205
Chapter 38—The Partially Sighted As A Driver	206
Chapter 39—Optical And Non-Optical Aids To Help You See	209
Guide To Optical Aids For The Partially Sighted	213
Guide To Non-Optical Aids For The Partially Sighted	216

PART X—SYMPTOMS AND COMPLAINTS

Chapter 40—Listing of Symptoms And Complaints	221
Blurred Vision	221
Night Blindness	222
Distorted Vision	223
Temporary Blindness	223
Central Vision Loss	223
Side Vision Loss	224
Light Flashes	224
Double Vision	225
Floating Spots	226
Light Sensitivity	226
Halos Around Lights	227
Pain in Eye	227
Headaches	228
Redness	229
Secretions And Discharges	229
Frequent Blinking	230
Change In Pupil Size	230
Small Lumps	231
Colored Spots On White Of Eye	232
Eyelids	232
Protruding Eyeball	233
Shrinking Eyeball	234
Eye Oscillations	234

GLOSSARY 235

FOREWORD

As we look back, it seems inconceivable that three years have elapsed since the idea for this book was spawned. It happened in the lobby of a dinner theatre where Neil Simon's "Gingerbread Lady" was playing. Herb Solomon's wife, Phoebe, an excellent actress, was appearing in the play. Walt Zinn, who had been a professional photographer in his younger years, was drafted to take publicity pictures of the players. We (including Walt Zinn's wife, Barbara) attended all the weekend performances during the twelve-week run of the show. Many topics were discussed between acts, and somehow, the conversation turned to writing a book on vision care.

We were both aware that the great majority of people are relatively ignorant on this subject. Because of that ignorance, we were disturbed and exasperated; many people were receiving less than adequate eye care without even realizing it. It was and is our hope that a comprehensive, easy-to-understand book will encourage people to seek out better professional services.

By the end of the run of the show, we had an outline, effervescent enthusiasm, a budding comradeship, and the painful realization that writing for lay people is no easy task. Concepts that we could easily express to other professionals, became as difficult to put into simple language as climbing the Alps.

We often argued like the "Odd Couple." It was necessary to perform a marriage of the minds combining our experience, background and writing styles into one palatable approach. Walt Zinn had the lighter writing touch; Herb

Solomon was a stickler for the minutest detail. We spent about twenty-five hours a week writing, discussing, rewriting, rethinking, and rewriting. Because of our mini-debates, respect for each other's talents and knowledge increased, in no small measure.

It was a significant learning experience for both of us. For example, the research relating to myopia control alerted us to facts which we put to use in our private practices. While writing the chapter on tinted lenses, we recognized that our approach (and that of our colleagues) in prescribing tints had come under the influence of patient demand and optical manufacturer's promotions. Worse still was the shocking discovery that the public was being grossly misled and "sold" on potentially harmful tinted lenses via advertising.

Those of you who are into astrology would contend that we enjoyed the provocative mental stimulation of writing this book because we are both Geminis. Perhaps so. But, whatever the reason, we certainly did enjoy it. We hope the reader, too, will find it provocative, informative, and gain a fuller appreciation of the many facets of optometric vision care.

        Walter J. Zinn, O.D.
        Herbert Solomon, O.D., D.O.S., F.A.A.O.
        Glencoe & Niles, Illinois

Part I

YOUR VISUAL WORLD

CHAPTER 1

WHAT'S YOUR VISION ALL ABOUT?

The odds are 99 to 1 that you need eye care now or will need it in the future. Your life style, your occupation and even your life depend on good vision. You get more information about the world through your eyes than all your other senses combined. Yet, vital as it is, you tend to take your vision for granted. What do you really know about your eyes and how you "see?" Why do you have two eyes instead of one or three? How do you see colors? Why must the eyes work together? What can a cataract do to your vision? Are your "sunglasses" doing you more harm than good? How do you know if your child has good vision?

You probably know less about your vision than you do about acupuncture, vitamins, and diets. If you are the average person, you worry much more about your teeth than about your eyes, probably because toothaches can be painful and teeth can fall out. Well, eyes don't usually fall out and poor vision doesn't always hurt, although it may be disguised as a headache, fatigue, or avoidance of near tasks (the child who "hates" to read). Does it make any sense to concern yourself less with your vision?

Most parents will anxiously drag a child to the dentist twice a year to check for cavities, poor bite, protruding teeth, etc. These same parents are not aware that neglecting a child's vision may lead to grave consequences such as poor schoolwork, limited job choices later in life, or even blindness.

In carrying the teeth versus the eyes argument to its most

ridiculous conclusion, we offer an example: The state of Illinois requires a checkup by a dentist before a child can be enrolled in school. Would you care to guess what is required for vision? The general health form filled in by the pediatrician carries the single word "EYES" along with height and weight, etc. In no way is the pediatrician capable of evaluating the child's vision, and if he was completely honest about it, after the word "EYES" he would fill in—"Yes, two of them."

It's certainly nice to have good teeth, but when was the last time you learned anything with yours? Obviously, Illinois feels that if a child can chew gum, the child is ready for school. Other states are more enlightened and require a comprehensive eye examination for school enrollment.

Consider this quote: "The demands upon our eyes in our days have greatly increased over those made by our ancestors. . . . The demands upon school children's eyes have been excessively increased in the last fifty years."

Does this sound appropriate? It was written in 1894, eighty years ago, by Dr. St. John Roosa, Professor of Diseases of the Eye and Ear, New York Medical School and Hospital. It was written *before* electric lights made reading for many hours into the night a general practice; before television and movies; before cars were driven at high speeds; before fifteen years of schooling was common (add many more years for advanced degrees); before the era of technological miniturization and micrometer tolerances.

All of these activities are dependent on vision, and as far as the natural evolutionary development of the eye is concerned, most of them are highly artificial.

Is extreme sharpness of vision necessary to milk a cow? Do you need binocular vision to stomp on grapes to make wine? Does a crossed or a "lazy" eye keep you from planting corn?

There is no doubt that modern civilization puts demands on our eyes for which they were not designed. The authors have seen many patients with symptoms of discomfort, headaches, doubling of vision, etc., which were directly related to the patient's occupation or life style. There is not too much we can do about the way our modern technological society is run. (We may long to return to those simpler bygone days, but few of us would be willing to give up all the conveniences, benefits, and comforts we enjoy.) Modern civilization is here and we are stuck with it, for better or worse. But, we must carefully watch the abuse our eyes are taking in the process!

Small deficiencies in clarity, differences in the way the two eyes see, poor focusing ability, or lack of stereoscopic vision, may not matter too much in a slow agrarian society; but they will play havoc with an individual's effort to cope with the present environment, school or occupation.

What you are about to read is a comprehensive treatment of the many problems which can beset your eyes, how they can be alleviated, or, how, at least made more tolerable. The information is geared to cover not only all of the questions lingering in your mind, but to help you make new and fresh discoveries.

CHAPTER 2

DO YOU SEE WHAT YOU ARE LOOKING AT?

Your off-hand answer to this question would be, "of course." A couple of examples and a few minutes of thought might change your mind. Look at the illustration below. What do you see?

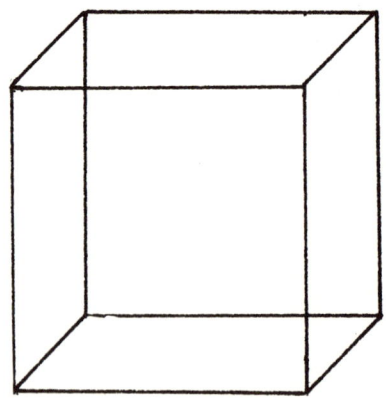

Do you see what you are looking at?

This is the common Necker cube. By looking steadily at it, the figure will flip-flop. The front surface will become the back surface and vice versa. The changes are spontaneous and not under your conscious control. Try as you will, you cannot keep the box in one orientation.

You might think this example unfair because it is an illusion. Indeed it is—a *visual* illusion as contrasted to an *optical* illusion. (The difference is explained in Chapter 6.) Far from being an isolated incident, the Necker cube only dramatizes that all vision must make certain decisions as to size, distance, motion, etc.

Notice, please, that we use the term "vision" and not "sight." Sight is the input from the eyes, while vision is the resulting perception you experience in the brain. Really, this Chapter should be titled "Do You Vision What You Are Looking At?" but grammar forbids it.

Let's clear up the difference between vision and sight. Take a stroll through any art gallery and look at the impressionistic paintings and sculptures. The confusion (and/or frustration) you may experience occurs when you cannot figure out what it is. You certainly see it, the colors, lines, forms, etc., but you cannot interpret it visually. You have no stored image in the brain to make recognition possible. This is the crux of the whole problem—vision is *interpretation* of what the eye sees.

Do you really know what you look like? Sure, you see yourself in the mirror all the time, but it's not the way others see you. (We are using the word "see," although you should think "vision.") The image in the mirror is reversed. Your right eye looks directly at your reflected right eye, while if another person was standing there, it would be opposite the left eye. This accounts for one of the reasons you look strange to yourself on television or in home movies.

The difference goes deeper than that, however. "Beauty is in the eyes of the beholder," is an *almost* correct saying. If you substitute the word "brain" for "eye," it might not sound as romantic, but it would be more accurate. Assuming normal sight, the image the eyes receive is about the same for most people. What the brain does to interpret that image makes the difference. Experience, culture, and emotions all enter into what you visualize.

We don't know, however, if everyone visualizes colors in the same way. Even discounting those people with known color vision problems, does red look the same to everybody? Color is very much a part of our vision and perception. Do you think you would be comfortable eating a blue orange (besides having to call it a blue)? A green steak? Probably not. Even more intriguing, you tend to visualize objects in their true colors although they may not be that way physically. If you look at an orange orange through green glasses it will still look orange. (Mull that over.)

You will now begin to realize that seeing and vision are not the same, are not automatic, and are subject to many variables. In fact, except for basic innate functions, meaningful vision is a learned process which takes place in the brain from stimuli generated in the eye. If we add nearsightedness, farsightedness, astigmatism, poor eye coordination, disease, color deficiencies, or a host of other anomalies, we may indeed ask: Do you see (vision) what you are looking at?

CHAPTER 3

THE EYE

Without a doubt, the eye is our most important sense organ, accounting for about 80% of our awareness of the environment. Moreover, it is the only sense organ without any distance limitation. Touch and taste are obviously contact senses; smell and hearing have a limited range and lack specific localization. Yet, you can look up at the night sky, locate and see a galaxy so very far away that the light from it may have taken thousands of years to travel through the universe. Without much fuss, your eye can also localize and see objects a few inches from your face with great detail.

Your eye can see in very bright sunshine and in almost total darkness, covering a brightness range of 10,000,000 to 1. It can see a rainbow of colors, and, with its partner eye, can see in depth. It can detect the movement of a single leaf on a giant oak and can track moving objects with uncanny precision.

However, the eye can't do all these things by itself. Ultimately, the remarkable feats are accomplished by the eye's commander, advisor, and controller—the brain. Before discussing that part of the story, let's take a closer look at the structure and functions of the various parts of the eye.

THE EYEBALL is a sphere about an inch long, crammed with many specialized parts. In cross-section it looks like this:

The eye

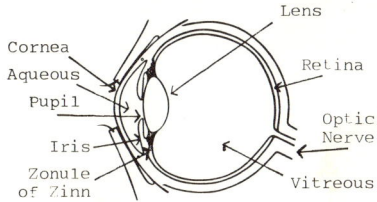

THE CORNEA is a transparent tissue covering the front of the eye much as a watch crystal covers a watch. (Contact lenses are fitted over the cornea.)

THE IRIS is a thin circular curtain which is the colored part of the eye. A person's eye color depends on the amount of pigment in the iris; light blue has the least amount and dark brown the most.

THE PUPIL is a hole in the center of the iris. It is black because the inside of the eye is dark. The size varies with the amount of light entering the eye, i.e., it gets smaller with increased light.

THE LENS is a transparent, semisoft material about one-half the size of a dime. It can change shape to focus on objects at different distances from the eye. It is held in place by threadlike fibers called the Zonule of Zinn (alas, not named after one of the authors of this book). The fibers are connected to the ciliary muscle. To focus at a close object, the ciliary muscle contracts, loosening the fibers' tension on the lens and allowing it to bulge. This increases the optical power of the eye.

As the lens ages, it loses some of its pliability and cannot bulge as much. This is called presbyopia (aging eyes), and is the reason people in their 40s tend to need reading glasses.

The inside of the eye is filled with fluid. The small area between the cornea and iris contains water-like aqueous humor; the larger area behind the lens is filled with a jelly-like vitreous humor. The varying amount of aqueous fluid in the eye determines its pressure. An increase in this pressure may result in glaucoma.

THE RETINA is the lining at the back of the eye where the image is formed. It is composed of specialized light-sensitive cells, various typical brain-type cells, and a network of arteries and veins. A comprehensive study of the retina is outside the scope of this book. We will deal with those aspects which are related to various visual problems.

In cross section, the retina is a formidable complex system of interconnected nerve cells. What is strange is that the

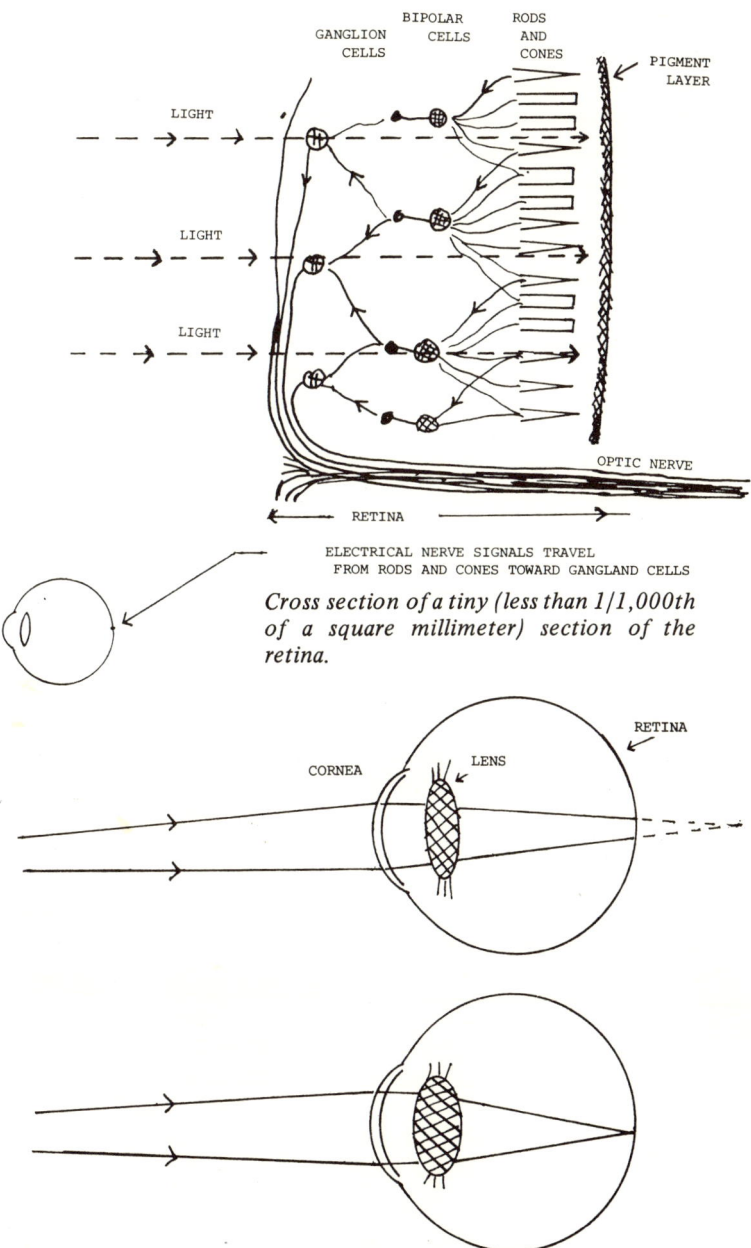

Cross section of a tiny (less than 1/1,000th of a square millimeter) section of the retina.

ACCOMMODATION. Light from a nearby object comes to a focus "behind" the retina causing a blurry image. This triggers a command signal from the brain for the lens to bulge and focus the image onto the retina.

retina is functionally inside-out. Light has to travel through all the layers before it can strike the light-sensitive cells. This topsy-turvy arrangement is probably due to the embryological development of the eye as an extension of the brain.

If you recall a bit of basic biology, the light receptor cells are the rods and cones. The rods are much more numerous than the cones and more sensitive in low illumination. The cones can distinguish fine detail and color, but require brighter light. Therefore, it's difficult to discriminate colors in dim light.

The cones are packed quite close together in the center of the retina in a region called the *macula*. In the center of the macula is a tiny depression, the *fovea*, which is the area of sharpest sight. Since the macula is responsible for detailed seeing, it has been called the seat of our civilization. When you "look" at something, you turn your eyes so that the light rays are focused precisely on the fovea. Keep this point in mind when we discuss the problems of crossed eyes and "lazy" eyes.

In all, there are about 130,000,000 light-sensitive cells in the retina, 120 to 125 million rods, and 6 to 6½ million cones. Most of the cones are packed into the macula which is only 1/20th of an inch in diameter. The very tightest concentration of cones is in the fovea (147,000 per square mm.), which is one of the reasons it has the keenest sight. The fovea enjoys two other advantages. There is very little overlying tissue to block the light rays (remember that the cones are at the bottom), and each cone has an almost direct nerve line to the brain, while many rods in the periphery have to share a common line. It's like having a hot-line telephone compared to having a party-line hookup.

The much more numerous rods are distributed throughout the retina, the number getting fewer at the extreme edges.

The tiny size of the macula severely limits your area of best vision. This simple illustration will prove it to you. If you close one eye and hold the page about eight inches away, you can only clearly read the pennant. To read the words in the other pennants, you must shift your gaze to point the fovea there.

There are always comparisons made between the eye and the camera. It is a reasonable comparison until you reach the

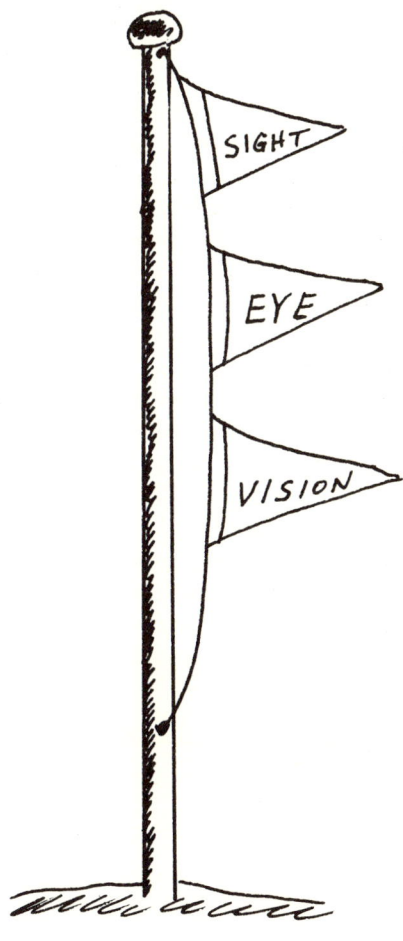

retina, which is totally different from film. The most obvious difference, of course, is the retina's ability to view many images in rapid succession, while a sheet of film can only record a single image. But, it goes much deeper than that. Photographic film simply responds to light. While there are some retinal cells which signal the brain when a light is turned on, others signal when the light is turned off!

Most of the cells are organized into recognizing very discrete patterns. For instance, some will only signal a black vertical line on a light background; others a black horizontal line; still others for in-between meridians. There are some groups which signal borders—but only borders in a particular orientation. Other populations of cells respond to movement, but each group to only one direction of movement. While all this is going on, there are the additonal responses to colors which are sent to the brain. You now begin to grasp the complexity of the retina.

Approximately one million nerve fibers carrying electrical impulses generated by the retinal cells (estimated at about one billion bits per second), leave the eye via the optic nerve. This area, about 1/20th of an inch in diameter, is devoid of visual cells and is, therefore, blind—the normal blind spot of the eye.

Want to find out for yourself? Stare at the X with the left eye closed. Start at about sixteen inches and slowly bring the page closer. At a certain distance, when the image of the face falls on the blind spot, the face disappears. Bring the page a little closer, and as the image falls on light sensitive cells again, the face reappears.

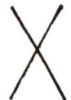
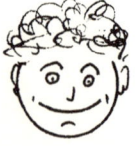

The blood supply to the retina also enters at the location of the blind spot. The vessels divide and branch out to cover the entire retinal surface. This is the only place in the body where blood vessels can be examined in their natural state.

Six muscles attached to the outside of the eye, constantly move it to keep the image on the fovea. These movements are so habitual and normal that generally you are not even aware of them. The teamwork among these muscles must be precise and critically accurate. Furthermore, they must match the movements of the other eye. Since there is no connection between the muscles of the two eyes, the matching is done by nerve impulses from the brain.

Not actually a part of the eyeball, but quite important, are the eyelids. They protect the eye from foreign substances, close to shut out light, and by regular blinking, keep a layer of tears over the cornea. This is vital to maintain the transparency of the cornea.

CHAPTER 4

WHY TWO EYES?

Since most of the organs of the body are paired, you might have taken your two eyes for granted. If you stop to think about it, you might decide that with two eyes you get a wider field of view to the sides. True, but to have a really terrific field of view, wouldn't you be better off with one eye on a tentacle atop the head for seeing all around? Wouldn't it be nice to have the ability to see behind your back? There is evidence of a prehistoric animal which had an eye with a 360 degree panorama. That would seem to be a tremendous evolutionary advantage. Yet, nature abandoned that route in favor of our present system. Why?

Actually, by itself, a very wide field of view is not all that great. It's good for noticing movement and general shapes, but it's very poor for seeing in detail. (Try threading a needle out of the "corner" of your eye.) Seeing movement is adequate for a frog since it merely triggers reflex action, but, for us it is important to know what caused that movement. Is it a rhinoceros charging, or only the overhead shadow of a bird? To make this vital decision we must see it in detail. Why can't we see in detail over the entire field of view? Very simply, the limited size of the brain.

As you will recall from the previous chapter, the area of best sight is the macula, some 1/20th of an inch in diameter. The flood of nerve signals from this tiny area alone, keeps a large part of the brain occupied with interpreting the visual meaning. If the entire retina had the sight property of the macula, it would require a brain the size of a football field to back it up, a huge head to house it, and a neck to support it. Our vision is actually a compromise. To the sides we have a reasonable field of view without much detail; at the macula we have a very limited view with marvelous detail.

It would be possible though, to have this combination with just one eye bulging out of the center of the forehead. This is impractical, however, because the eye would be very susceptible to injury. (A punch in the eye would be disastrous.) So, the eye has to be placed within a bony vault for maximum protection. If you put your mind to it, you could come up with many possible arrangements for the eyes, including one fore and one aft. But, there is a very distinct advantage to frontally-placed eyes with overlapping fields of view—it's depth perception.

Before you say, "Is that all?," remember that nature thinks so much of stereoscopic vision that a very elaborate system is involved to produce it. The retina is divided almost exactly in half, with the nerve fibers from the outer half connecting to the brain on the same side, while the nerve fibers from the nasal side cross over and connect to the opposite half of the brain. This seems like a curious arrangement. The crossing over is not strange, however. You know that the right hand is controlled by the left half of the brain, and so on. The curious thing is that half the fibers do not cross over. Herein lies part of the secret of depth perception.

Because the eyes are about two and one-half inches apart, each retina receives a slightly different image. You can readily see this if you place your finger eight inches in front of your nose, close one eye at a time and watch your finger change its apparent position. Deep within the brain there are special cells which match the offset images from the two eyes to yield the sense of depth.

There is another way the brain uses the two eyes for depth information. The nearer an object is, the more the eyes have to turn inward to keep it centered on the macula. The amount of turning is signaled to the brain for evaluation.

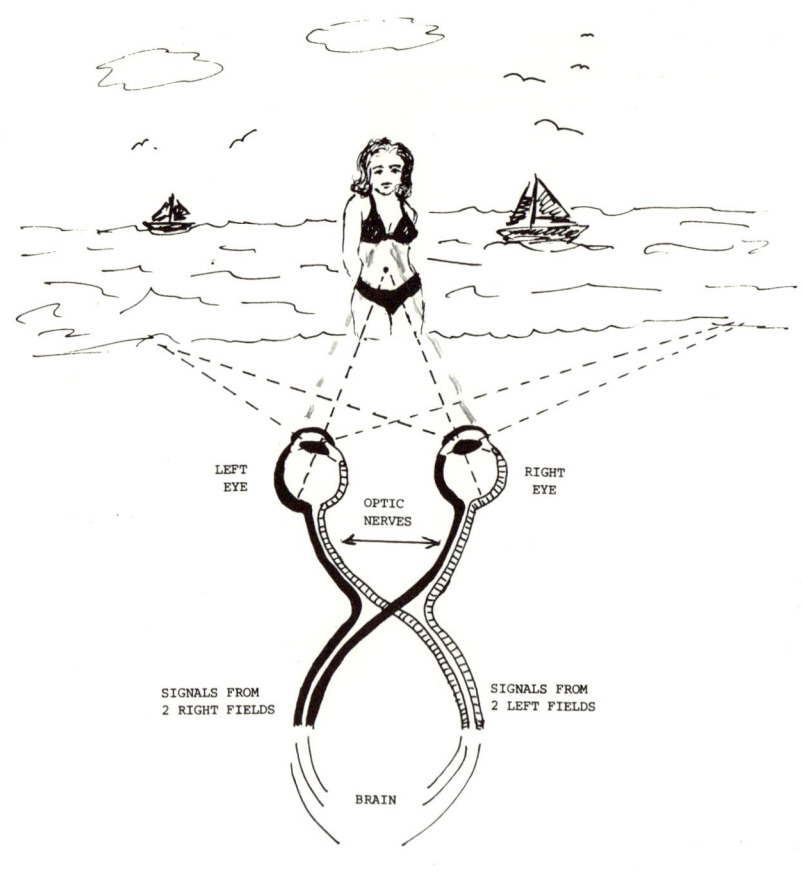

A diagramtic view showing the crossing over of nerve fibers.

This, incidentally, is the way an optical rangefinder works.

Is depth perception all that important for survival? It is difficult for us now to reconstruct exactly how much advantage it conferred on our ancestors. Perhaps it gave our tree dwelling forefathers and foremothers an edge when they swung from branch to branch; they knew exactly where in space that next branch was located. Grasping and picking up objects is much simpler with depth perception. Whatever the reasons, nature labored millions of years to perfect it, so let's enjoy it.

As with any system, the more complicated it is, the more potential it has to go wrong. To appreciate the full value of depth perception, very precise and intricate alignment of the eyes is necessary. Horizontally, the alignment must be within a few degrees; vertically, even less. If the six muscles controlling each eye cannot point the two eyes at the same spot within this range, the stereoscopic effect will be diminished or lost. The very narrow range of the vertical alignment explains why people with one eye sighting slightly higher than the other experience difficulties, and may even see double. You can appreciate the importance of testing this faculty during an eye examination.

CHAPTER 5

"I SEE," SAID THE BRAIN

If you've followed along so far, you understand that we have two eyes sending billions of nerve signals through the optic nerve to the visual cortex of the brain. Here's where the real magic takes place. Somehow (and science is just beginning to unravel the mystery), the brain interprets these signals into a stable, colorful, three-dimensional world *out there*.

You realize, of course, that the brain does not "see" the tiny, two dimensional, upside-down, constantly shifting, distorted image on the retina. No light gets to the brain at all; it only receives patterns of electrical nerve impulses from which it must extract meaning. Volumes have been written, and are being written, on this complicated mechanism we call vision. For the purposes of this book, we will confine ourselves to some of the more intriguing highlights.

The fact that the image on the retina is upside-down seems to puzzle some people as to why we don't see that way. But, remember that the brain is not looking at the back of the retina. It constructs the visual world so that down is where your feet are normally planted, and up is towards the sky.

A more difficult idea to reconcile is that the eyes are in almost constant motion, yet we see the world as a stable entity. Besides constantly shifting around to view various parts of a scene, the eyes also make slight jerky movements called saccades. How can the brain get any meaning from a constantly shifting image? Surprisingly, these movements are necessary for vision. The visual cells in the retina respond best to changes, with a rich outpouring of signals to the brain—changes in brightness, changes in direction, changes in orientation, or changes in speed. Without these changes, the rods and cones would quickly lose their sensitivity.

Try this experiment. Stare at any object and make a strong effort to keep your eyes perfectly still. It is very difficult to do, but if you can manage it, notice how parts of the scene will begin to fade away. Chances are that you will make a slight eye movement, because the brain will not easily tolerate loss of vision.

Scanning is vital for recognition. When you see an object for the first time, the brain will try to match it section by section with stored memory images. Curves and angles are very important as major clues. (You will recall that vast numbers of retinal cells respond to borders and lines.)

Think back a moment. The first time you looked at a new automobile model, you had to look carefully and at length so that the brain could absorb the new configurations. The eyes made rapid scanning movements, lingering the longest on the most modified parts. You hardly looked at the tires, but did glance several times at the redesigned bumpers and grill. Once this information was absorbed and stored by the brain, you recognized that particular automobile at perhaps a single glance, or so it seems. Actually, the eye made a few rapid movements which usually followed the original sequence. Again, the angles and curves are very important.

By the way, have you ever wondered how the brain receives a separate image from each eye, but you see only one object? Hold your thumb up at arm's length and sight across it (both eyes open) at a distant target. Do you see two thumbs? In all, you see three things—the distant target plus two thumbs. Why? The answer is tied up with the mystery of depth perception. Apparently, the special brain cells which have the ability to combine similar objects located within a given range and angle from the eyes into a single sense of depth, also inhibit the two individual images from being seen.

In the case of your thumb, by looking past the position of the two thumb images, they are outside the operating range of those brain cells. Hence, no inhibition of the two images.

So far we've been talking about a still life object. Suppose we now complicate matters by having the object move. The images shift around on the retina *just as they do when the eyes move.* How does the brain know the difference? Suppose you are riding in a train. How does the brain decide if the telephone poles are on a treadmill, or if you are moving? The brain must deal with inputs from other sources in the body (such as your neck muscles, legs, etc.), and also make reasonable guesses based on past experience. Most of the time the decisions are correct, but sometimes the brain is fooled into a visual illusion.

You *can* make the world shift by introducing an unusual type of eye movement. Place your finger on the lower lid and gently push the eyeball (close the other eye). Now, the world moves because the brain has no experience at integrating the finger's push. We know of no experiments, but perhaps if this were done a few hundred-thousand times, the brain would learn to compensate for it and the world would not move.

You can tell the size of an object by the size of the image on the retina, right? Wrong. There is very little relationship. A person's face at twelve inches away may cover the entire retina, while the same face across the room may only cover five percent of the retina. Yet, you don't see the former as the face of a giant. The brain utilizes what is known as size constancy. If you know the size of an object, you will "see" it that way no matter what the size of the image on the retina. The evolutionary survival value of this faculty can be easily understood. Imagine moving very close to a pussycat, only to discover it's a sabertooth tiger! Or chasing that cute little cub, only to come face to face with a huge grizzly bear! Size constancy is a very necessary faculty for maintaining order in our visual world. Sometimes, though, as you will find out in the next chapter, it can lead to false conclusions.

Have you ever been annoyed by the flickering of a

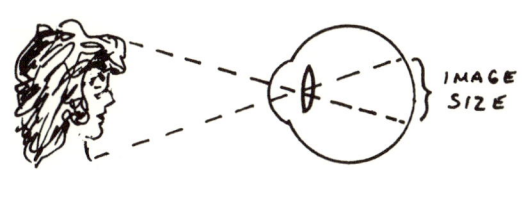

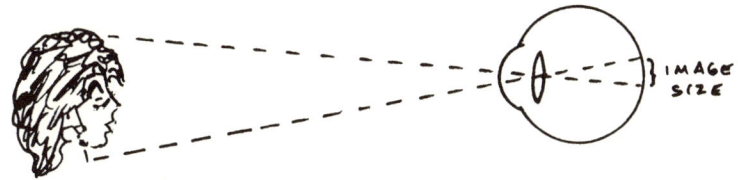

SIZE CONSTANCY. *Though the image on the retina changes size depending on the distance of the object, the brain visualizes it in its true size.*

fluorescent light? These tubes work by flashing on and off sixty times per second. Normally, it looks like a steady light because the retina has a slight persistence of vision. This means that you see the flash of light slightly longer than the actual physical flash. At about thirty-five flashes per second, the persistence overlaps enough to make it look like a steady light. For a bright light like a fluorescent, it takes about fifty flashes per second to look constant. When the tube becomes old or defective and the flash rate decreases, the individual flashes become noticeable flickerings. Because the rods are more sensitive, these flashes are sometimes bothersome to your side vision. This has probably happened to you—there seems to be a flicker, but when you look directly at the light (with the central cones), it looks steady. Feel assured that this is quite normal.

The remarkable brain doesn't even need a complete image to get vision. Just a few lines on a piece of paper will elicit visual meaning. Look at the drawing. Do you have any trouble "seeing" that it's a bird's-eye view of a man riding a bicycle, even in depth?

Still more remarkable, the brain doesn't even need a drawing. Just the word "elephant" conjures up a visual memory. However, if you don't know what a duck-billed platypus is, there is no visualization. How this visual memory works is not yet understood. But, it is fascinating. If we ask you how many windows there are in your home, you can visualize and count them. Even more interesting, you can visualize the windows from various angles without ever having looked at them that way!

This will give you some idea of the complicated workings that go on in the visual system *before* the brain can say: "I see!"

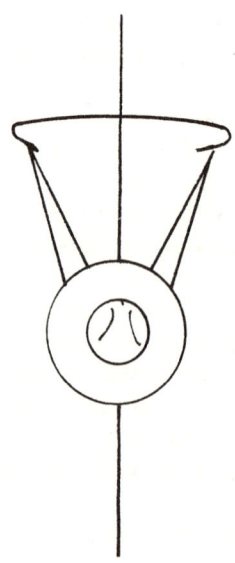

I see a bicycle rider.

CHAPTER 6

VISUAL ILLUSIONS

Let's get one point cleared up right away—a visual illusion is not the same as an optical illusion. An optical illusion is caused by an outside device, usually optical (hence the name)—a lens, a prism, or a mirror. For instance, a telescope produces an illusion of enlargement; a mirror (or reflection in water) may produce an illusion of an upside-down scene. One of the newer, more fascinating optical illusions is created with a hologram and laser which produces a life-like image in space.

But, a visual illusion is created within the visual system, not externally. It is the result of the brain's *normal* struggle to make sense out of the information it received from the eyes, information which is frequently scanty, unreliable and may be in conflict with information coming in from other senses.

You are aware from the previous chapter that the visual cortex not only extracts meaning from, but places its own interpretation on, the signals from the eye. Often there are several possible ways of interpreting the total flow of information into the brain. What it comes down to is that the brain must make a "best bet" to decide what you are looking at.

For example: Suppose that on a clear summer night you are looking up at the stars. Suddenly the star pattern begins to rotate like a giant pinwheel. The brain has only a fraction of a second to decide whether the heavens are spinning, the

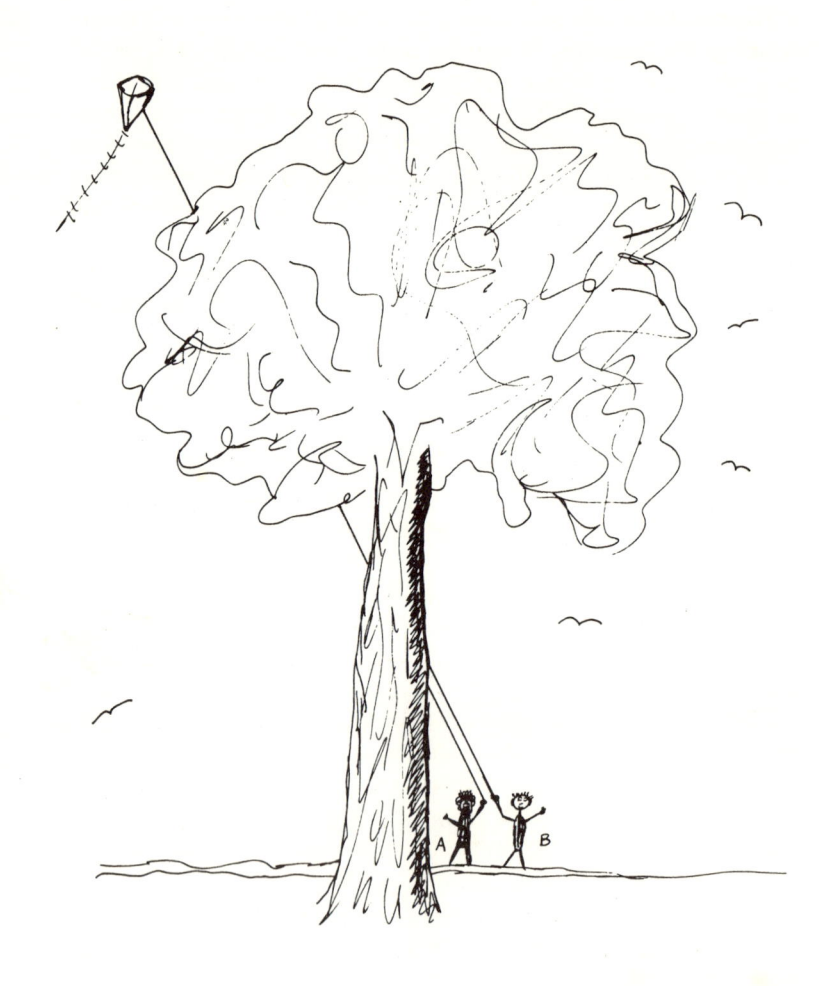

Which child is flying the kite? Check your answer with a straight edge ruler.

world is spinning, or you are spinning. The "best bet" is that you are whirling (perhaps you are sitting in a swivel chair).

We can turn this situation into a visual illusion by actually rotating the heavens. It can be done (and is done routinely) in a planetarium where the projected star pattern can easily be made to whirl. When this happens, the brain "best bets" that you are in a spin and you will grasp the arms of the chair to keep from falling off. Even though your other senses may tell you that you are sitting still, the visual sensation will completely overwhelm them.

As a kid you almost certainly spun yourself around and around in a room, and when you stopped, the room seemed to spin in the opposite direction. Here is a plausible explanation. Suppose you are spinning to the right. The visual cells responsible for seeing objects moving from right to left become fatigued from the constant input. This causes a drop in their signal strength to the brain. When you stop spinning and the input ceases, the signals drop to almost zero. However, the visual cells sensitive to the *opposite* (left to right) motion, are "fresh" and though receiving very little stimulus, will overpower the signals from the weary cells. The brain, therefore, interprets the room moving in the opposite direction. Yet, there is still a puzzling aspect—the room both moves and remains in the same place. Go ahead and try it.

The fatique of motion-direction cells also explains the loss of your sense of speed after driving at 55 miles per hour for a long time. Surely you have felt as if you're barely crawling along an exit ramp after turning off an expressway. Unless you watch your speedometer very carefully, this visual illusion will cause you to go dangerously fast.

Most common visual illusions, some of which are pictured here, are artificially created by a drawing which is in itself an artificial creation. All pictures and drawings make use of visual clues to induce the brain into thinking that you are looking at a real object with real depth.

By putting perspective in drawings, such as converging lines and various sized objects, the illusion of a real scene is evoked. But, by altering the normal perspectives, false illusions are created. "Impossible" objects are created this way.

Here's an interesting situation: If you look at the ellipse and the circle, you know that the circle is too big to fit through the ellipse.

But, by adding a few additional lines, it is a basketball arcing towards the distant basket and certain to go through. What's more, you see the basket as circular and not elliptical.

Try this experiment. It's a beautiful way to convince yourself of size constancy as discussed in the last chapter. If you have a strobe flash gun, look directly at it and flash it. You will see an afterimage, the size of which will change depending on the distance you are looking at! Hold a sheet of paper ten inches from your face and the image is small; look

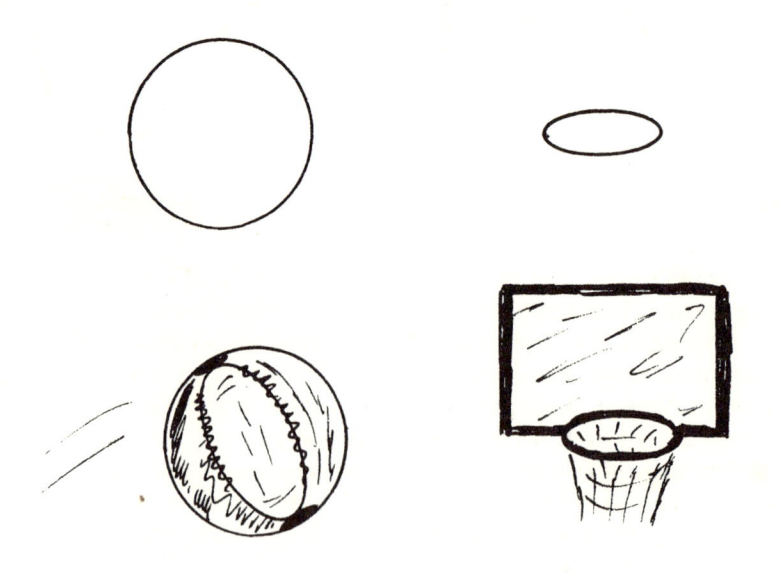

Visual illusion

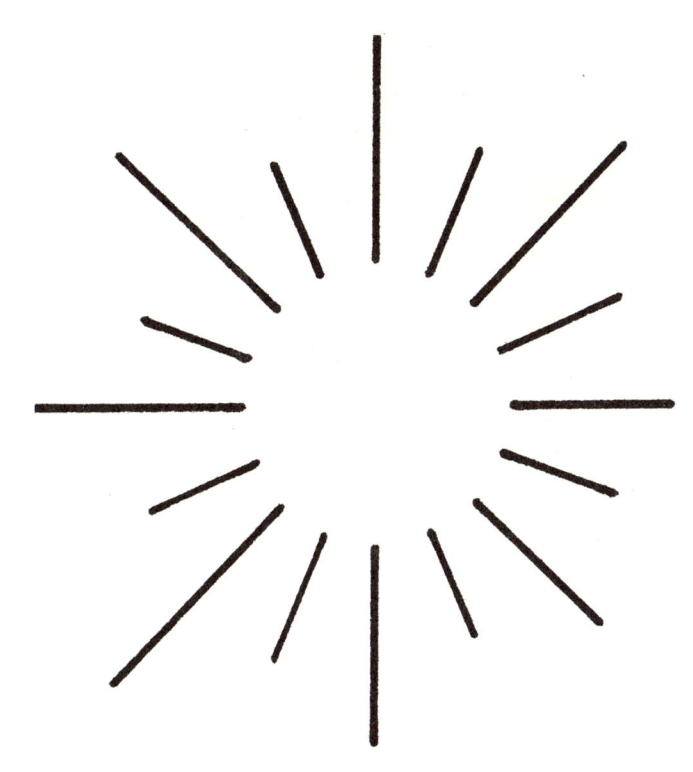

There is a distinct impression that the area within the lines is brighter.

across the room and it enlarges dramatically. (You can prolong the afterimage by blinking.) In other words, the brain interprets the same retinal image size, as an object of various sizes, depending on where the brain thinks it is. (If you don't have a flash gun you can do the same thing by staring at a light bulb for a count of fifteen.)

Understanding this will help you to understand the moon illusion. When you drive along at night, the moon seems to follow along. (The sun does the same thing during the day, but it's not as easy to watch.) Even though you intellectually know that the moon is a quarter of a million miles away, the

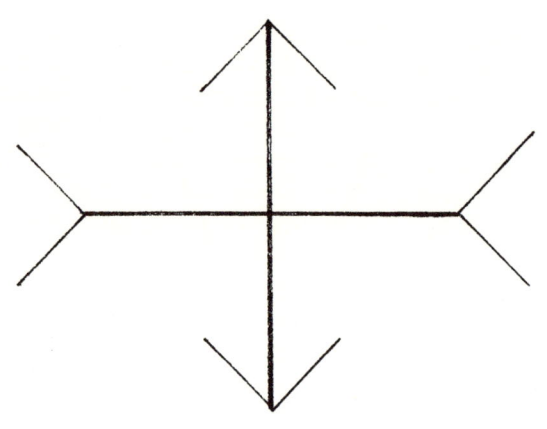

Is the horizontal line longer than the vertical line?

retinal image makes it appear as a large object, perhaps a few miles away. But, here is a problem for the brain. While other objects a few miles away of the same apparent size (a large building or a hill) are soon passed up, the moon is still in the same place. This could only be possible if, indeed, the moon was moving with you. But, because the brain blithely makes this assumption, that is what you see.

The size of an object also influences your judgment as to how fast it is moving. The moon in the above situation, seems to move much slower than the fifty miles per hour you may be driving at. People who live near airports are quite convinced that giant 747s land at much slower speeds than the smaller airliners, even though their physical speed is the same.

The famous Necker cube is an example of insufficient information leading to a definite conclusion. There is no "best bet," because either one is perfectly plausible. So, the brain keeps trying each version alternately and indefinitely.

Naturally, the more detail in a scene, the easier it is for the visual system to choose the "best bet." Conversely, the fewer the clues the brain has to work with and the more assumptions it has to make, the more likely an illusion. That's why most of the illusions in real life occur at night under dim light conditions, particularly when there is motion involved. Any wonder most UFOs are reported at night?

You can understand why an airline pilot coming in for a landing on a foggy night may easily miscalculate the dim image of another airplane. Is it a large jumbo jet far away, or a small plane nearby? Which way and how fast is it moving in relation to him? Remember, apparent size will influence movement interpretation.

The occasional illusions we experience are the price we have to pay for a very flexible visual perception system. Retinal images are used to trigger a previously-stored image in the brain. This is much more efficient than having to laboriously study each scene every time it occurs. But, sometimes it will trigger the wrong stored data—presto, an illusion.

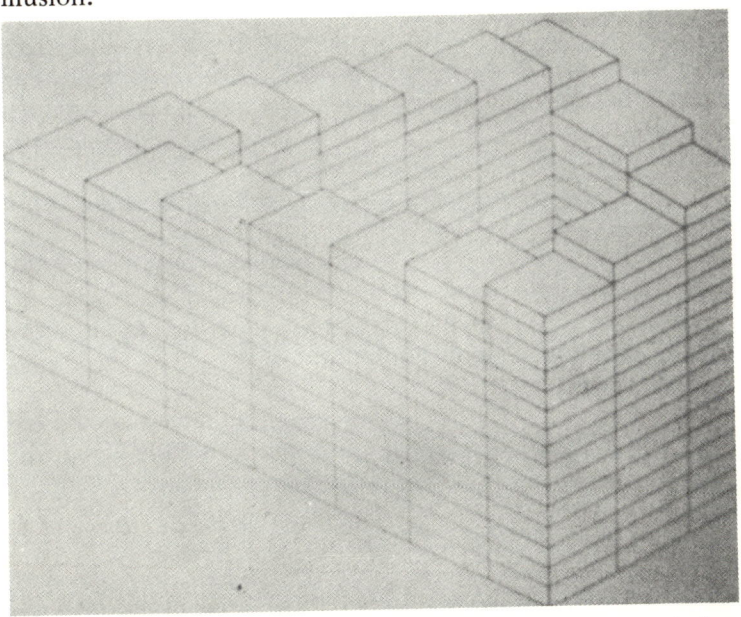

A newly invented staircase which will find its greatest use in large government buildings. Bureaucrats can walk up or down all day long without getting anywhere. Of course, it's an "impossible figure" illusion.

CHAPTER 7

COLOR VISION

To be absolutely technical about it, if you study the physics of light, there is really no such thing as color. There are only various wavelengths of light which give rise to a sensation of color in our visual system. You might, if you were given to puns, call it a pigment of the imagination! Yet, in practical terms we do see in colors like birds, bees, and many other animals which also have this remarkable gift. Your dog, however, does not see in color, so he'll be just as happy watching TV in black and white.

There are a number of theories as to how color vision works. None are completely satisfying because we just don't have all the answers. But, it is fairly well established that there are separate receptors in the cones of the retina for each of the primary colors—red, green, and blue. By mixtures of these three in various combinations, we see all the colors. This is known as normal trichromatic color vision.

For example, a yellow bikini will stimulate both the red and green receptors to signal the brain in a code which the brain recognizes as "yellow." Purple is a mixture of red and blue, and so on, with every possible hue included. White is produced from a mix of the three primary colors.

The mixing of colored lights to produce another pure color, is a very unique property of the visual system. Musical notes cannot be mixed to obtain a third pure note. But, colored lights mix completely and there is no way to see the separate wavelengths. Yellow is the most striking example. It is made up of red and green, but you see no trace of either.

People who have difficulty recognizing colors are commonly said to be color blind. Yet, the term color blind is very inaccurate. Only very few people are so totally color blind that they see the world as a black and white photograph. This very rare condition usually accompanies other vision defects such as nystagmus (rapid eye oscillations) and poor sight.

Generally, the problem is a color deficiency which makes certain colors or certain shades hard to recognize. About one in twelve men have some form of color deficiency, while only one woman in two hundred suffer from this disturbance. It is a genetic defect, always affects both eyes, and does not change appreciably during a lifetime. There is presently no known cure. The commonest type of color problem is the eye which uses all three primary colors, but in wrong proportions. Such people require brighter colors for recognition. Pastels are particularly affected. During times of fatigue or stress, even the bright colors may be misjudged. If you have one of these people around the house he or she is always setting the color TV with too much red or too much green to suit you.

Another type of color deficiency is the person who uses only two of the three primary colors. Such an individual will be "red blind," "green blind," or in extremely rare cases, "blue blind." The red blind individual does not see reds and oranges as the normal person does. These hues look dark gray or even black. A flashing orange or red traffic signal could look the same. All purples look like shades of blue because the red part of the mix is not seen. To the green blind person, reds, oranges and greens all look the same and even have the same brightness. If he goes hunting, a fellow hunter in a bright red jacket will not show up well against the green background. It seems to us that a color vision test would be advisable before issuing a hunting license.

All is not hopeless for the color deficient person, however. Some interesting work is being done with filters and tinted contact lenses which often help this individual to tell colors apart. Even though the colors won't be seen as the normal person sees them, differences between the various hues will be distinguishable.

It is possible to acquire color deficiencies as the result of disease or aging. If it is caused by a disease, it will most likely only affect the diseased eye. Successful treatment of the disease may restore both the sight and color vision.

Various chemicals and medicines may have a temporarily disturbing affect on color vision. For instance, barbiturates used as sedatives may cause changes in yellow-green vision; excessive use of caffeine from coffee, tea or cola drinks, will alter the sensitivity to almost all colors. Huge doses of vitamin A may cause your world to become yellow.

Because color is used extensively in the classroom, color vision should be checked at an early age. Pity the green blind boy who is told by the teacher that all the nouns are on green cards and all the verbs are on orange cards. He's lost before he begins.

Another reason for early detection is to help in choosing a career. Occupations such as painters, chemists, interior decorators, engineers, etc., rely heavily on good color vision. The individual should be aware of the potential difficulties he or she might encounter.

Part II

HOW YOUR EYES SHOULD WORK AND WHAT CAN GO WRONG

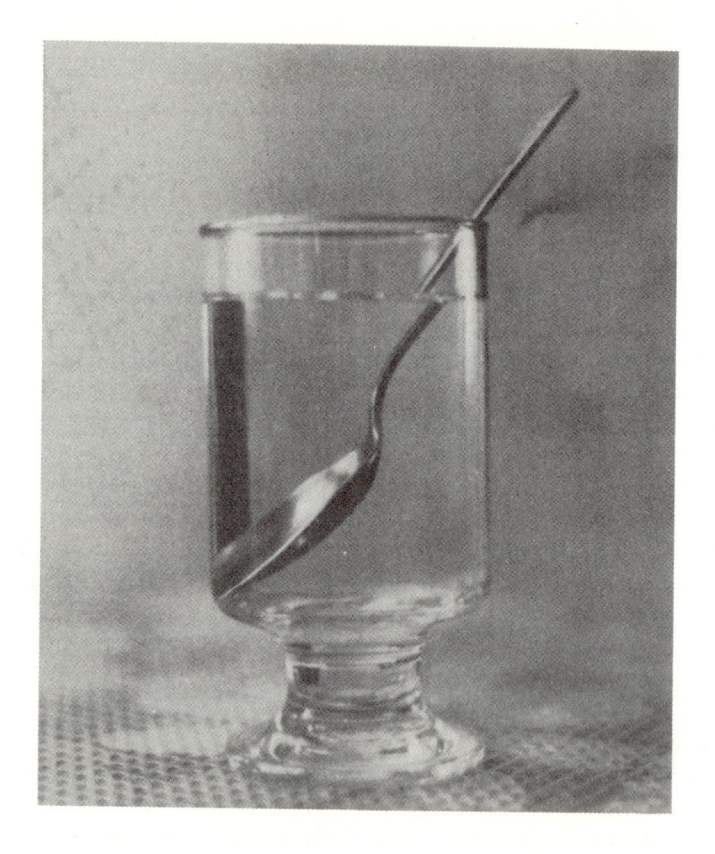

Normal focusing and eye movements

CHAPTER 8

NORMAL FOCUSING AND EYE MOVEMENTS

The long chain of events which ultimately result in vision, of course, begins in the eye. Nothing can happen until an image is formed on the retina. For the brain to get the most information, the image must be sharp and clear, with crisp borders and angles. The clarity of the image is known as visual acuity and that is where the familiar 20/20 comes in.

What do those numbers really mean? Without getting technical, the distance acuity is measured by using letters of a certain size at 20 feet. The top number is the distance at which you *can see* the letters; the bottom number is the distance at which you *should be able to see* the letters. For instance, 20/40 means that you see at 20 feet that which you should be able to see at 40 feet. 20/100 means that you see at 20 feet what you should see at 100 feet.

For a few minutes, let's forget that the eye is a living organ and only consider it as an optical system to focus the outside world onto the retina. The word "refraction" is indispensable in this discussion, so let's define it.

Light rays normally travel in straight lines. Refraction means that the light rays are bent when they travel from one transparent medium into another of a different density. The simplest way to understand this is to place a spoon into a glass of water and look at it from the side. The spoon seems to be broken at the surface of the water. The reason is that the light rays going through the water are bent—refracted—more than the ones going through the air.

The eye has several transparent mediums of differing densities through which the light rays must travel to reach the retina. The greatest amount of refraction takes place at the front surface of the curved cornea which is much denser than the air. (By the way, have you ever opened your eyes under water and noticed that your vision is blurry? The water, being denser that air, alters the normal refractive power of the cornea and upsets the focusing balance of the eye.)

The lens is another major refractive body. But, while the cornea has a fixed contour, the lens is able to modify the amount of refraction by actually changing its shape. It is, in effect, a variable focusing system to bring light rays from an object to a sharp focus, regardless of its distance from the eye.

Here's how it works. When you look at something farther away than 20 feet, the lens maintains its minimum curvature and least bending power. When you look at something closer, the lens will increase its refractive power, to bring the light rays to a focus. The closer the object you're looking at, the more the lens must curve. This lens focusing is called accomodation and is controlled by the brain. A blurry image on the retina starts the action.

A very important point is that the brain signals both eyes simultaneously and equally. The two lenses cannot work independently.

If the amount of the refractive power of the eye exactly matches the length of the eyeball, a perfectly focused image is formed. Being a living organ and not an assembly-line product, there are many possible variations in the eye's refractive parts. A small change in the curvature of the cornea, or a difference in the length of the eyeball of as little as 1/75th of an inch, can throw the image out of focus. You may wonder if there are any eyes that have a perfect focus.

Assuming that we are lucky enough to have a sharp image on the retina, we must be sure that the focus is on the right spot. The eye must be able to keep the image centered on the fovea for best sight. This is no simple task when you realize that the eye is constantly moving and what you're looking at is often moving.

The brain is constantly engaged in a hunt and find game. It does this with a steady stream of signals to the six external muscles of the eyeball. The signals are fed evenly to both eyes so that they move together. Normally, they cannot work separately. (With practice you can learn to pat your stomach and rub your head, but no amount of practice will enable you to move one eye up and down while the other moves back and forth.)

But, hold on, things get even more complicated. There are two basically different types of eye movements. The first, in which the two eyes move in the same direction, i.e., to the right or left, or down. The second, in which the eyes converge, turn inward, to keep an object centered on each fovea. While the same muscles are involved in these manuevers, the task is different. Both types of movements occur simultaneously. As you read this, your eyes are sweeping back and forth while they are also converged.

Want to see convergence at work? If there is another person handy, hold a pencil about twenty inches in front of his or her nose and slowly advance the pencil towards the nose. The person is to keep watching the pencil; you will see the eyes converge, turn inward. A person with good convergence should be able to follow the pencil in to about three inches before one or both eyes will swing outward.

Looking at near objects requires both accomodation of the lens and convergence of the eyes. Evolution of our visual system has linked these two functions together, and the brain triggers both at the same time. A given amount of accomodation drags a given amount of convergence with it, and vice versa. It's economical for the nervous system, but leaves the visual system open to all sorts of problems which will be discussed in later chapters.

DISTANT
LIGHT RAYS

RETINA

LENS

SPECTACLE LENS

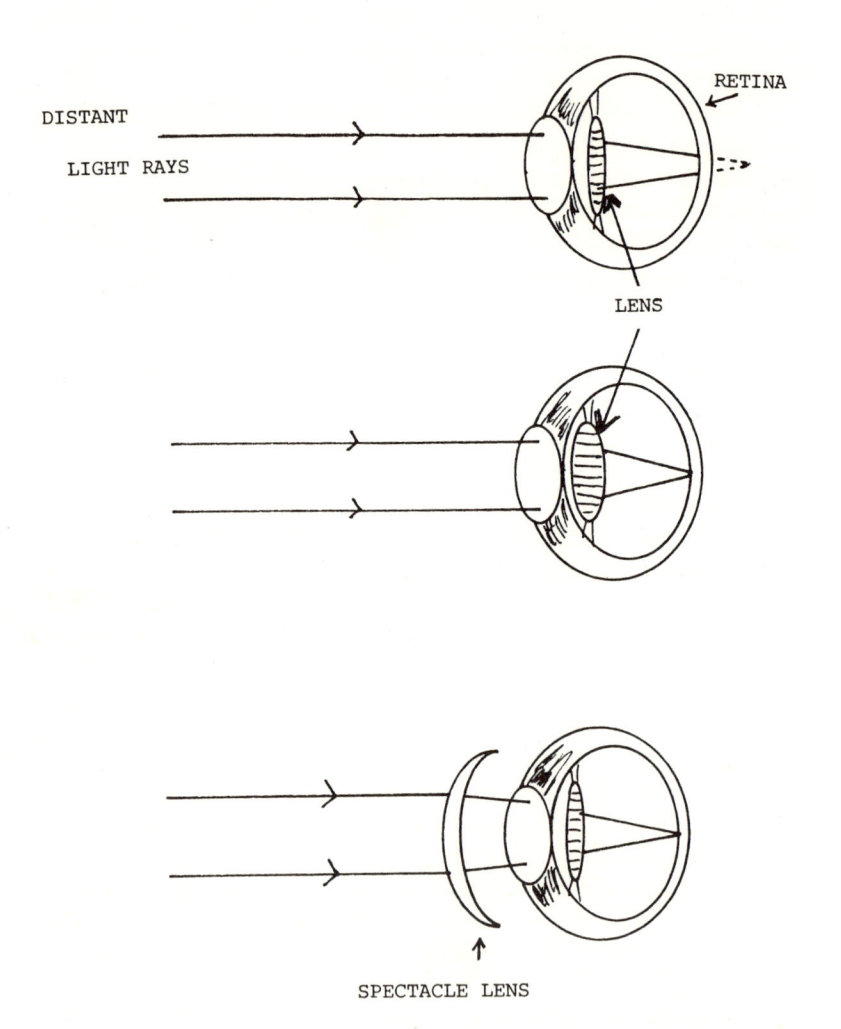

HYPEROPIA, FARSIGHTEDNESS. Light focuses "behind" the retina producing a blurry image. Accommodation by the lens within the eye compensates for moderate amounts. By means of a convex spectacle lens a clear image is focused on the retina relieving the accommodation effort.

CHAPTER 9

COMMON SIGHT DISORDERS AND CORRECTIONS

There are four common refractive problems of the eye. A refractive problem exists when the image is not properly focused on the retina. This occurs in hyperopia (farsightedness), myopia (nearsightedness), astigmatism and presbyopia (aging eyes).

The hyperopic or farsighted eye is essentially too short for the refractive power of the eye. Hence, the light rays from a distant object would theoretically come to a focus behind the retina. Actually, this can't happen since the retina is in the way. If you have ever set up a movie or slide projector, focused the picture on the screen, then moved the screen closer, the picture will be out of focus. That's exactly what happens with the hyperopic eye—the retina is too close.

Here's where a little maneuvering takes place. The blurred image on the retina looks the same to the brain as the blurred image a normal eye sees when looking at something close up. So, the brain signals the lens of the eye to increase its power and bring the focus forward onto the retina. (From the previous chapter you recall that the lens is capable of changing its shape to increase the refractive power of the eye.) While this system is designed for seeing up close, the hyperopic eye makes use of it for distance seeing. It works, too, as long as the amount of farsightedness is not excessive and the lens remains flexible. Hyperopic people can generally see clearly at a distance. There is one major flaw, however. Since part of the lens focusing is used for distance seeing, less

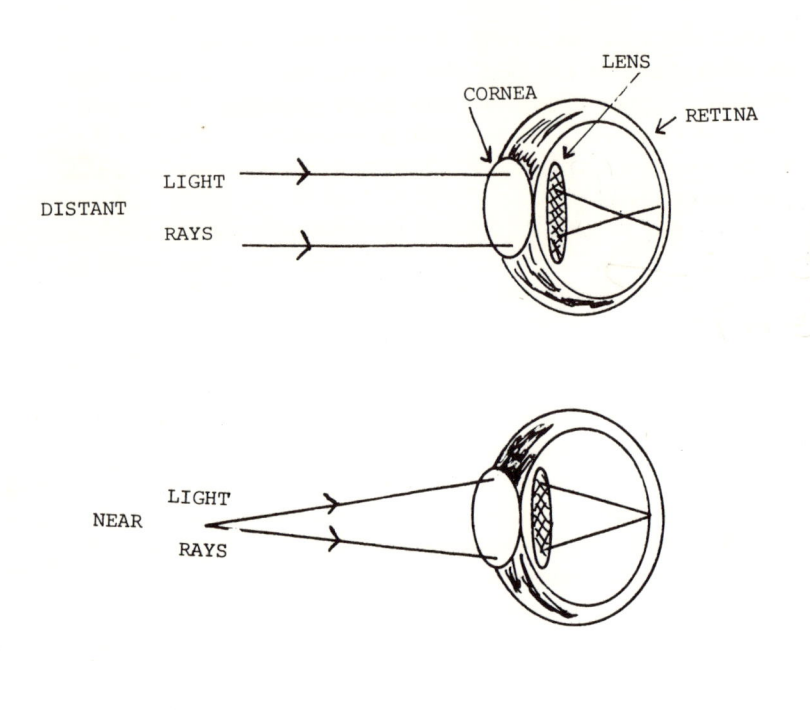

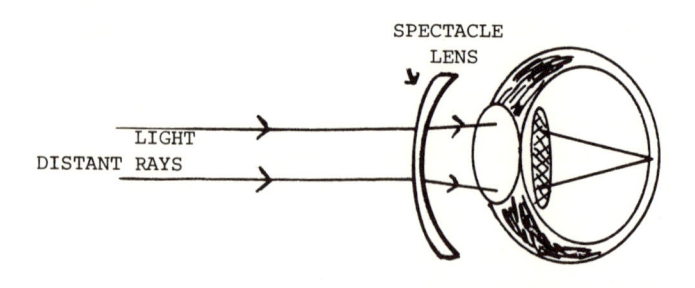

MYOPIA, NEARSIGHT<u>EDNESS</u>. Light from a distant scene focuses in front of the retina then spreads out to produce a blurry image as in the photo. Only a nearby scene will focus on the retina. By means of a concave spectacle lens a distant scene is focused clearly on the retina.

is available for close seeing. If this person is required to do a lot of reading or detailed close work, the extra strain may produce fatigue, headaches and other problems. Even without a lot of reading, as the person gets older and the ability of the lens to alter its shape is lessened, the distant vision will also become blurry.

If the eye is *very* farsighted the distance vision, even in young people, will be affected. Hyperopia does not mean an eye which necessarily sees well far away, but one that merely sees better far away than close up. In the case of high hyperopia or if symptoms are present, the optometrist will prescribe glasses or contact lenses (convex lenses). Many times it may only be necessary to use glasses for close seeing.

The myopic or nearsighted eye is too long for its refractive power. The light rays come to a focus in front of the retina, then spread out to form a blurry image (like moving the movie screen back). There is no way for the eye to clear the image, since any action by the eye's lens will only bring the image forward and even further from the retina. The nearsighted eye can see things clearly if they are reasonably nearby. These people will frequently squint in order to see better. The narrow opening between the lids helps to sharpen the image. The optometrist will prescribe glasses or contact lenses (concave lenses) to enable the person to see distant objects clearly by moving the focused image back onto the retina.

There are many theories for the development of myopia and for the fact that it seems to be getting more prevalent. We do know that nearsightedness generally shows up in a child of primary grade age and continues to become progressively worse during the growing years. Because these are the years of intense reading and close work in school, near point tasks are the prime suspect. (See Chapter 31, Control of Nearsightedness.)

Astigmatism is a common disorder, but a difficult one to explain. If any of the refracting surfaces of the eye are not symmetrical, the light rays will not come to a clear focus point in either the front or the back of the retina. Looking at a tiny point of light, an astigmatic eye would construct it on the retina as a blurry streak. The culprit is usually the corneal surface (although it could be the lens and even possibly the retina). Instead of being round like the surface of a balloon, it is slightly oval as when a balloon is squeezed. This causes an unequal focusing power and, hence, distortion. You can get the idea by looking into an oval teaspoon and noting the distortion caused by the shape.

The same kind of distorted image is formed on the retina. But, while it may be blurry and indistinct, the person is not aware of the distortion because the brain has learned to compensate for it. Therefore, an interesting thing happens. When the optometrist corrects this defect with cylindrical lenses in the glasses, the person will see clearly, but often complain of objects being tilted and out of shape for a few days, until the brain learns to see properly. If not corrected, astigmatism will often cause headaches and eye strain. Frequently, it is an additional complication to hyperopia and myopia.

Presbyopia, or aging eyes, catches up with most people in their 40s. The first symptoms are difficulty in reading small print, threading a needle, having to hold a newspaper at arm's length, and complaints that a reading light is not bright enough.

As the lens of the eye ages, it gradually loses its flexibility to bring near objects into clear focus. Farsighted people are affected at an earlier age because they use part of the focusing to see far away. A succinct description of presbyopia would be: The brain is willing, but the lens is weak and the arms are too short. The brain continues to send signals to the lens to accommodate it, but the lens cannot respond as it did when it was younger. The optometrist will prescribe glasses (convex lenses) to compensate for the reduced ability of the lens to focus. These can be in the form of reading glasses or bifocals.

While it is possible for both eyes to have the same exact

refractive condition, it doesn't happen too often. If they differ greatly and are not corrected soon enough, a host of other problems including amblyopia and/or crossed eyes may result.

Presbyopia

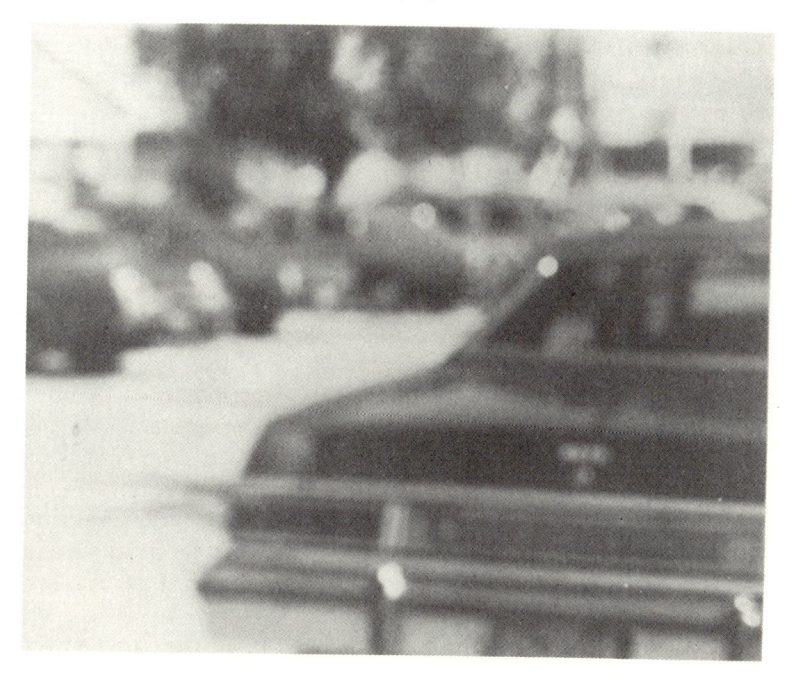

Part III

THE EYE EXAMINATION

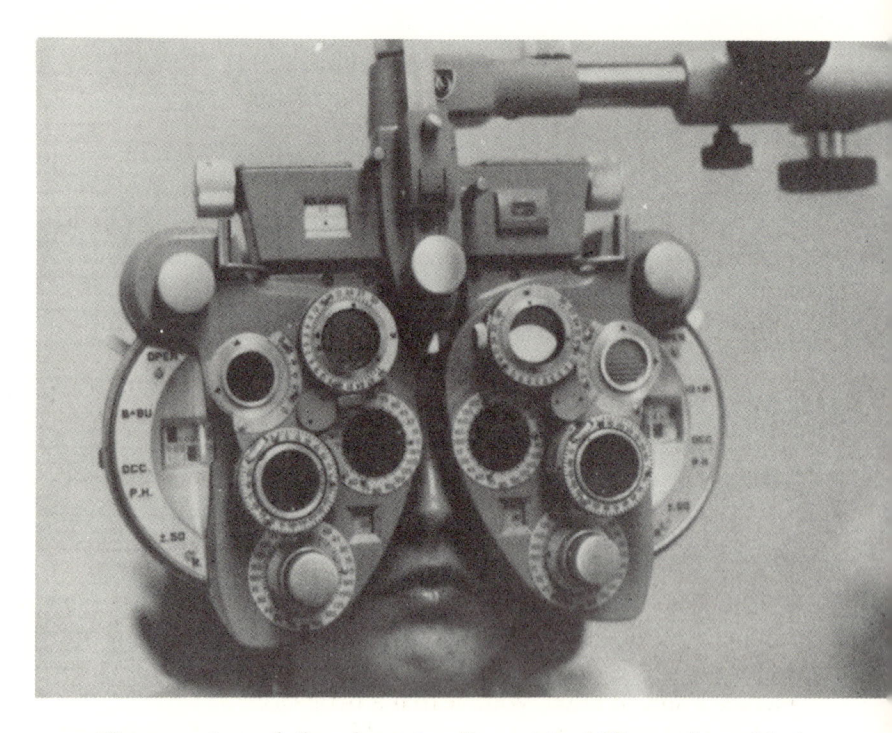

Close-up view of the phoropter. It contains billions of possible lens combinations.

CHAPTER 10

HOW TO CHOOSE A FAMILY OPTOMETRIST

Perhaps we should first ask: "Do you need a family optometrist?" If you're the kind of person who has a family dentist and a family physician, you should certainly have a family optometrist. But, it must be an *optometrist*. An ophthalmologist won't do since this doctor is, as you know, basically a surgeon concerned with diseases and injuries of the eye. If there is a need for such services, the optometrist will tell you. It's the same idea as your dentist telling you when you need a periodontist, or your physician referring you to an orthopedic surgeon. The optometrist is the general vision care specialist and is the one to consult when you have a vision problem. Sooner or later you will need eye care, so you might as well be prepared.

Choosing a family optometrist is about as easy or difficult as finding any other professional person to suit your needs. Here are a few tips to help you avoid the most obvious mistakes and to make your search a little easier.

As a starting point, you could ask your friends and neighbors for a recommendation. Ask someone whose opinion you respect. There is no guarantee that you will like the optometrist, but it's certainly worth investigating.

Better still, call the state optometric association for a list of optometrists in your area. Each state has its own optometric association which is affiliated with the American Optometric Association. To be a member, the optometrist has to adhere to a strict code of ethics and behavior in dealing with the patient. Any complaints are usually resolved in pretty quick order. If there are many complaints, the optometrist is dropped from the association. The association will be listed under the name of your state, i.e., Kentucky Optometric Association, California Optometric Association, etc.

If the above two suggestions are not feasible, you can, as a last resort, look in the yellow pages under "optometrist." However, finding an optometrist this way is like picking a winner at the race track by closing your eyes and sticking a pin into a name. You might come out lucky, but the chances are not good.

To increase your chances, by all means avoid box or display ads. An ethical, competent optometrist has no need to advertise. In fact, if he belongs to the professional association, he is prohibited from advertising. Look for a simple listing. When you do find someone, on the initial phone call ask him or her if he or she belongs to the state association. Of course, this is no guarantee that you will find the perfect optometrist, but it does improve the odds.

Specifically, you should look for an optometrist in private practice who will treat you as an individual and is interested in your problem. The office should be pleasant and clean, the equipment should be modern. When you read Chapter 12, The Vision Examination—What It Must Include—you will be in a better position to judge the testing procedures. If there is anything you don't understand, ask. The optometrist should discuss what your problem is and how he or she hopes to solve it. If the answers are short or uncommunicative, get yourself another doctor.

Considerable advertising is done by optometrists and optical departments of various emporiums and department stores. Remember what we said about advertising, and stay away. Most likely, the advertising optometrist is incompetent and under the direction of a lay person. These lay people have found that they can make an easy dollar by merchandising glasses like merchandising shoes or washing machines. The optometrist is used as yet another type of salesperson, albeit a sophisticated one. But, even if the optometrist is very competent, he or she cannot take the necessary time to give you a complete examination because time equals money. His or her employer is not concerned with your vision or eye health (despite what they cleverly say in the ads). Their only interest is making money, and lots of it. Since advertising is quite costly, they must operate on a high volume to pay for it. So, if you are foolish enough to go there, you'll get pushed in and out in a hurry. The examination will be cursory and the diagnosis can easily be faulty.

All professional fields have people who are only out to make a quick buck. In the case of these optometrists, it's easy to tell who they are—they advertise themselves. The number of optometrists involved is relatively small, but unfortunately for the health and welfare of the unsuspecting public, they are most visible. Some states have wisely outlawed this type of practice. We agree wholeheartedly with such action and suggest that other states do the same.

Contrary to this sensible approach which protects the public, the Federal Trade Commission in its bureaucratic wisdom has declared that advertising, and particularly price advertising is needed to insure lower costs for glasses. Suddenly, advertising is supposed to be the great panacea in the eye care field. This same FTC has been battling against false advertising of over-the-counter drugs for many years.

Unregulated price advertising might conceivably lower the cost of glasses by a few dollars, but the cost to the patient/consumer in unreliable eye care would be much more. With the apparent blessing of the FTC, "bait and switch" tactics in the eye care field will flourish throughout the land. Although in most states there are laws against "bait and switch," the record of successful prosecution is generally dismal. Clever advertising bears little relationship to truth and many people will be enticed by the seeming "bargains."

Of course, with the knowledge you will gain from this

book, you will avoid all of these pitfalls. When you find an optometrist you can live with, stick to him or her. Over the years he or she will become familiar with your eyes and vision rendering any unusual changes readily apparent.

And, for heaven's sake, tell your friends about your optometrist; then they won't have to go through the same search you did.

CHAPTER 11

THE "DROPS" MYTH

Somehow, the myth has flourished that a vision examination requires "drops." The time has come to expose this silly myth because "drops" actually reveal very little about vision. Their main use, on occasion, is to aid in the diagnosis and treatment of certain diseases and/or injuries. (Sometimes they do aid in determining the refractive status of the eye.)

What are these mysterious "drops" anyway? Simply drops of any of several liquid chemicals. Instilled onto the eye and absorbed through the cornea, they act on the tiny muscles of the iris to dilate (enlarge) the pupil. Some of the chemicals will paralyze the focusing mechanism of the eye, as well. The avowed purpose of the dilating drops is to enable the doctor to look through the pupil into the eye for possible abnormalities. IT IS ALSO EASY TO LOOK INTO THE EYE IN ITS NORMAL STATE.

The pupil is merely the opening through which light enters the eye and through which you look out to see the world. Albeit, it's only a few millimeters in diameter, you can see a wide panoramic scene.

Looking through this same normal-sized pupil *into* the eye, the optometrist can see most of the internal features. Think of it as a knothole in a fence—when you're close enough, you can see virtually everything on the other side. If there are symptoms of disease, or if the center of the pupil is blocked by a cataract, it may then be advantageous to use drops to enlarge the pupil.

The key point for you to understand is that inspecting the inside of the eye is *only one* of many, many tests which must be performed to determine the state of an individual's vision. Rather than guaranteeing the very thorough examination that you expect, the use of drops may be a hindrance to an accurate diagnosis. When the effect of the drops has worn off, a complete examination must follow. Some of the visual activities which have to be investigated, i.e., focusing and muscle harmony, are so altered by drops that the results are uselessly distorted. Since a reading problem, for instance, may be intimately tied to those functions, how can they be tested and analyzed if they are paralyzed? The sensible approach is to deal with the eye and visual system in its normal state, not in an abnormal, drugged condition.

The promiscuous use of drops can be harmful in two ways. The first results from the chemical action of the drug itself. In susceptible people, there is the possibility of a glaucoma attack. In some children, one of the agents often used, atropine, may even cause systemic and allergic reactions. The second possible harm rests not in the drops themselves, but in the procedural method of those using them. Very frequently, the doctors who use drops indiscriminately, skip the important functional vision tests. In that case, you're getting a very poor, abbreviated version of an eye examination. Some doctors insist that young children can only be examined by first paralyzing their focusing. It can yield useful information in some situations, however, we feel that more valid results can be obtained without the drops.

When the eyes are drugged, it is impossible to accurately determine binocularity, muscle balance, focusing ability, or any of the other dozen factors which could be resposible for a vision problem. Since at least twenty-nine out of thirty people seeking professional help have a vision problem (not a disease), these tests are indispensable.

If you have ever gone through the drops routine, you know what it's like. Someone puts drops on your eyes; then you sit around for an hour or two. Of course, you realize that your eyes are not being examined during this time. You can easily spend a whole afternoon sitting around the waiting room before the doctor sees you for a few short minutes. A proper vision analysis cannot be done in a few minutes (with or without drops).

Why then do some doctors routinely use drops? A matter of training and habit. Ophthalmologists generally advocate drops for everyone; it's easy to comprehend the reason. They are trained to treat diseases and perform surgery on the eye. Therefore, they look for a disease in every case. If you are the one in thirty that falls into that group, it works out in your favor. But, if you are one of the other twenty-nine with a functional vision problem—too bad—your problem will receive only slight attention. The odds are definitely against you.

There is also a subtle psychological factor involved. A few doctors like to play God (you know the type), and by putting "magic" drops into your eyes, an image of the ancient witch doctor's esoteric omnipotence is created. You're supposed to be awed into silent devotion.

If there is evidence of disease or injury, dilating drops do have an important use as a diagnostic tool, much as X-rays are a diagnostic tool. But, neither should be used indiscriminately or routinely.

To sum up, for looking inside the eye, the drops are superfluous. They alter the normal state of the eyes and may hinder a correct diagnosis. They tend to encourage an incomplete examination. As with any drug, there are potential serious side effects. It is much more judicious to use drops ONLY in the few cases where the need is clearly indicated.

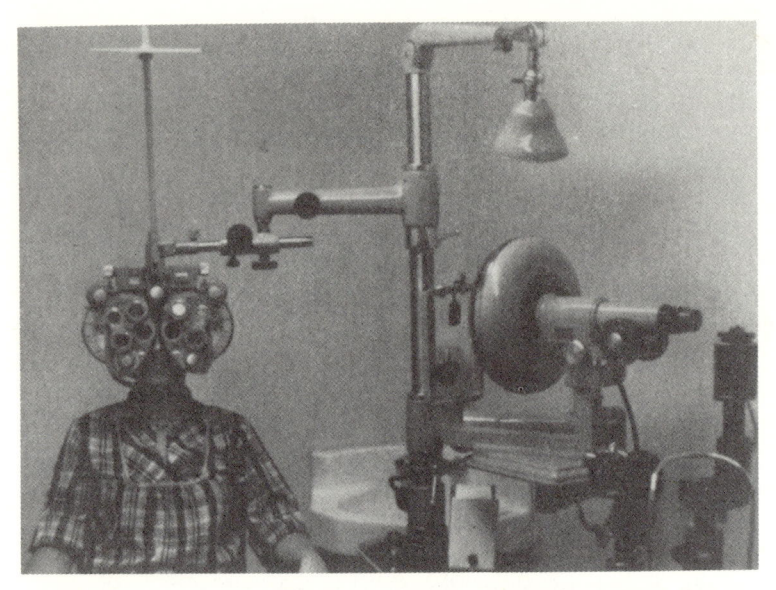

Examination of a patient in a typical optometric office. The ray gun-looking device to the right of center is used to measure corneal curvatures.

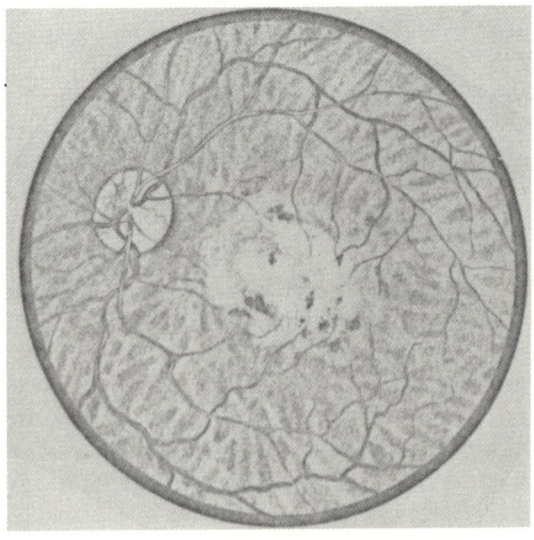

The retina as seen by the doctor through the ophthalmoscope.

CHAPTER 12

THE VISION EXAMINATION—WHAT IT MUST INCLUDE

Perhaps you are smart enough to have your eyes examined on a regular basis, or perhaps you wait until you have an eye or visual problem. Either way, when you put the phone down after making an appointment, do you have some notion of what the eye examination should include?

If it's your first examination, probably not. Even if you are an old hand at it, you may have only a general idea of what goes on. For your own protection, you should know more. The optometrist's ability to diagnose your problem is based primarily on an extensive vision examination, coupled with professional training and experience. Consequently, the examination must cover a wide range of tests; if it doesn't, the diagnosis and your prescription can be wrong.

Let's describe the general examination so you will be able to judge for yourself whether you are being properly cared for. We will describe what we consider to be the minimum tests and procedures (sometimes more are called for). The exact order is not too significant, but most doctors follow the sequence we will outline.

At first you will be asked a lot of questions, the key one being, "What is your visual complaint." We also want to know when your problem started, how often and when it occurs, its severity, and what you've been doing to try to get relief. Some of these questions may seem irrelevant, but they give the experienced optometrist some big clues toward a diagnosis.

When we ask about your occupation, we are not just being idly curious. You use your eyes quite differently as an accountant, a stevedore, a painter, or an auto mechanic. Your problem and symptoms might easily be tied up with your occupation. Furthermore, the final prescription must take your job into consideration.

"How is your general health?" and "Are you receiving any medical attention or taking any medication?" must be answered fully and carefully since many ailments can affect your eyes. Diabetes is a very prominent example; it can cause your vision to fluctuate wildly from week to week. Please remember to mention all medications you are taking. Many drugs have side reactions which affect the eyes ranging from a mild swelling of the lids to serious retinal complications. The best thing to do is prepare a list at home with all the names and dosages.

When the case history is completed, a series of screening tests is done. The point here is to find out how your eyes habitually function in everyday life. The functions which should be measured are:

1. The sight in each eye at far and near, both with and without your present glasses.
2. Your color vision.
3. How well your eyes work together at far and at near.
4. Intermittent suppression of either eye (stops seeing).
5. Your depth perception.
6. Whether the eyes move freely in all directions.

There are different instruments and methods for performing these tests; each doctor may have his or her own favorites.

The health of your eyes is the concern of the next series of tests. First, the lids and surface parts of the eyes are inspected for any sign of disease or injury. A simple but vital test is to check the reaction of your pupil to light. You may know that the pupils constrict in the presence of a bright light, but did you know that if they don't, or do so

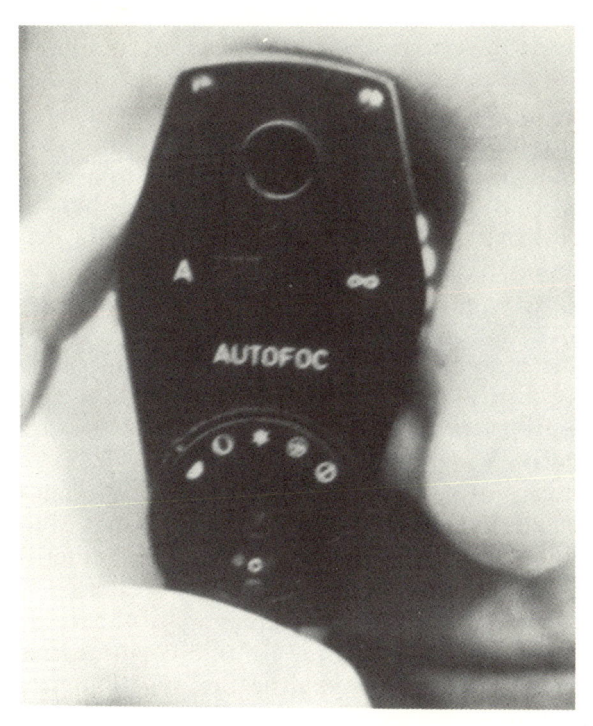

Patient's view of an ophthalmoscope which is used to observe the inside of the eye.

sluggishly, it may be the first symptom of a disease or neurological disorder? Or, it may indicate that you use drugs (either medicinal or harmful).

The optometrist will then turn his or her attention to examining the inside of your eyes with an ophthalmoscope. This instrument lights up the interior of the eye and enlarges the image. For a good view, we have to get within a few inches of your face, so we would appreciate it if you would avoid onion pizzas before your appointment. We examine the retina, arteries and veins, and the optic nerve entrance. The inside of the eye is the only place in the body where blood vessels can be seen in their natural state. It's not unusual, therefore, to spot the first signs of hardening of the arteries, diabetes, or hypertension in the eyes. We also look for specific eye diseases or abnormalities.

To examine the front parts of the eye, a slit lamp microscope is used. It sounds frightening, but it merely focuses a bright light on the eye and magnifies the view of the anterior parts about fifty times. It's also useful for monitoring the gradual progression of a cataract over a period of years.

If some serious problem shows up in your general health, or an eye disease is evident, it may be necessary to refer you to an appropriate practitioner. Happily, this has to be done infrequently.

Assuming your eyes are healthy, the optometrist will proceed to determine their refractive state. This simply means that we use lenses to measure whether you are nearsighted, farsighted, have astigmatism, or a combination of these. We do this by directing your gaze at a distant target while we shine the light from a retinoscope into your eyes. We are then able to analyze the motion of the lights and shadows on the retina. When this test is completed, we will ask the familiar question, "Which is better?" to subjectively fine-tune your visual acuity. Some patients are very concerned about giving a wrong answer. Just relax and tell it as you see it. You really can't make a mistake since all your answers are double checked. If you do make a mistake, it will not interfere with your prescription.

To conclude the refraction, we will show you a line of letters, half on a green background and half on a red background. By balancing the clarity of the two colored sides, the findings can be verified. To accomplish this, some doctors use polarized filters.

Once your sight has been corrected, tests must be run to determine how your two eyes will work together with these lenses. We will simulate all possible conditions and measure the limits of your eyes to turn inward and outward, the flexibility of the focusing system, and your reserve capacity to avoid fatigue. What does all this mean?

If you are a bus driver, we want to know if you can maintain clear, single vision hour after hour. If you are an accountant, can you keep the numbers from running together or blurring? If you are a student, can you easily change focus from the chalkboard to the reading material on your desk without tiring?

The final test will be to check the pressure of the fluid inside your eyes. This is the so-called glaucoma test. There are several ways of conducting it, none of which should cause you any discomfort.

The total examination can easily run to fifty or more individual readings, most of which are concerned with how your two eyes work together. The day is long since gone when all you had to do was call off a few letters on a wall chart. That might have been adequate in the horse and buggy age, but it is completely outdated in our modern, complex society. If your examination is not as all-inclusive as this, you are being taken.

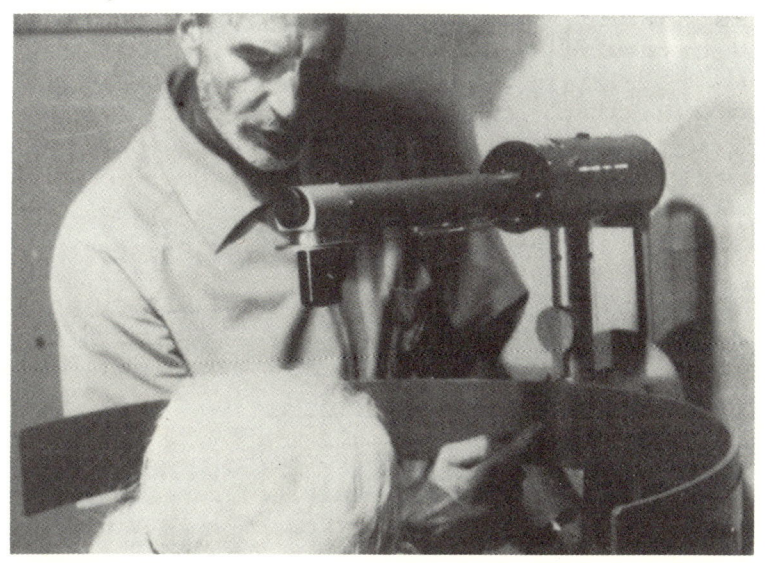

The field of view of each eye is tested with this instrument.

A COMPLETE OPTOMETRIC EXAMINATION CHART

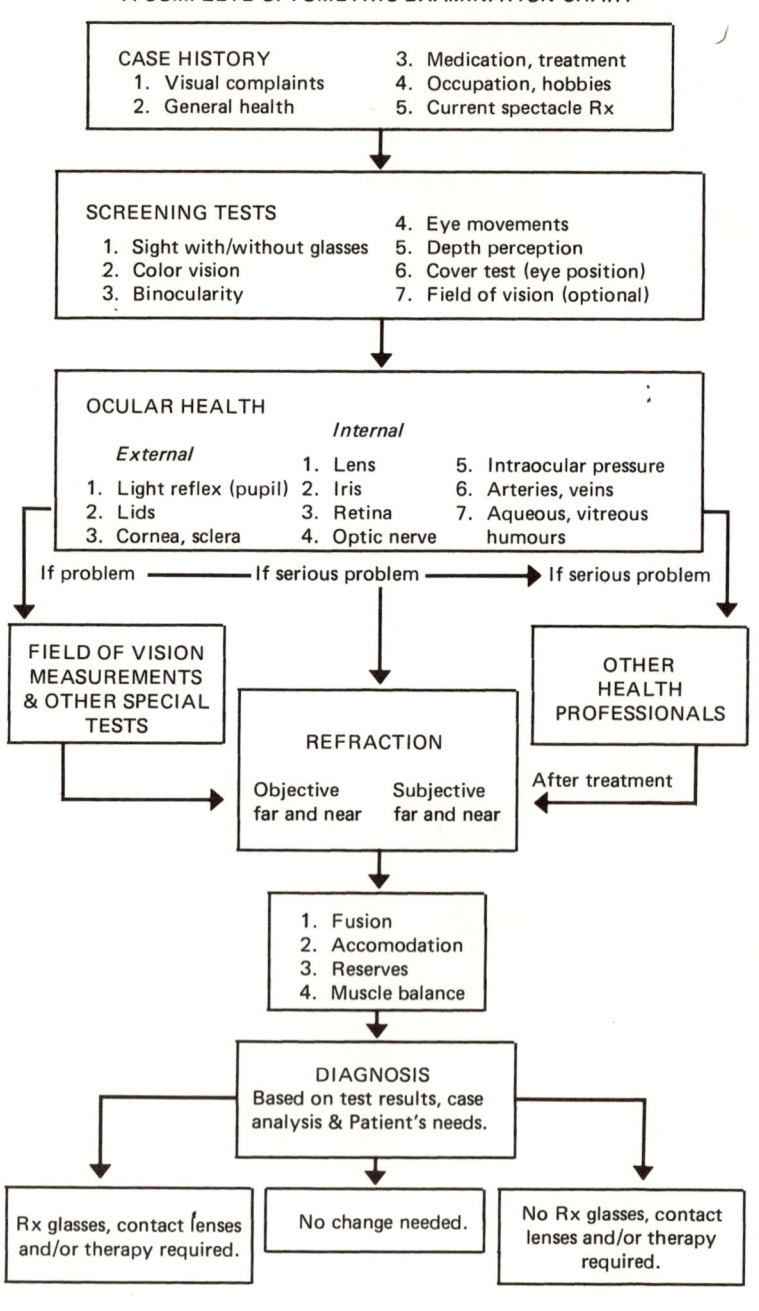

CASE HISTORY
1. Visual complaints
2. General health
3. Medication, treatment
4. Occupation, hobbies
5. Current spectacle Rx

↓

SCREENING TESTS
1. Sight with/without glasses
2. Color vision
3. Binocularity
4. Eye movements
5. Depth perception
6. Cover test (eye position)
7. Field of vision (optional)

↓

OCULAR HEALTH

External
1. Light reflex (pupil)
2. Lids
3. Cornea, sclera

Internal
1. Lens
2. Iris
3. Retina
4. Optic nerve
5. Intraocular pressure
6. Arteries, veins
7. Aqueous, vitreous humours

If problem → If serious problem → If serious problem

FIELD OF VISION MEASUREMENTS & OTHER SPECIAL TESTS

REFRACTION
Objective far and near
Subjective far and near

OTHER HEALTH PROFESSIONALS

After treatment

↓

1. Fusion
2. Accomodation
3. Reserves
4. Muscle balance

↓

DIAGNOSIS
Based on test results, case analysis & Patient's needs.

- Rx glasses, contact lenses and/or therapy required.
- No change needed.
- No Rx glasses, contact lenses and/or therapy required.

CHAPTER 13

SPECIAL TESTS FOR SPECIAL CASES

Occasionally, the routine examination will reveal or hint at some problem that requires further testing. Some of these conditions are not strictly vision problems, but since they affect the eyes, they should be investigated by the optometrist for possible referral.

The Dry Eye

The normal eye is kept moist by a thin film of tears on its surface. Most of these tears are produced by glands under the upper lid and are spread across the cornea with each blink. If the tear production is reduced for any of a variety of reasons, you will suffer symptoms of hot, burning dry eyes. In very severe cases, the cornea may dry, become cloudy and affect your sight.

We can check how much tear fluid you have by placing special strips of paper under the lids and noting the amount of wetness in a given time period. If the amount is moderately low, you can gain comfort by using drops of artificial tears. For a critical shortage, a soft contact lens may be indicated to keep the eye moist.

A dry eye can also result if the tear production is normal, but the blink reflex is missing. When this occurs, the tears cannot be spread across the eye.

Loss of Corneal Sensitivity

The next time you get a piece of dust in your eye resulting in pain and buckets of tears, be thankful that your system is working properly. The pain, of course, is a warning that something is irritating or damaging the cornea; the profuse tearing is an attempt to wash the foreign matter away.

In some rare instances, the cornea may lose its sensitivity. If you can't feel a foreign object rubbing the cornea, serious eye damage could result. It's quite easy to test for sensitivity with an instrument, or simply with a thin wisp of cotton. Total lack of feeling indicates a serious neurological problem.

Bulging or Protruding Eyes

We are not talking about people with naturally large eyes, but when one or both eyes give the appearance of *becoming* larger. It doesn't really mean that the eyes are getting bigger, but rather that they have started to protrude. If both eyes become more prominent, the "frog-eyed" look, chances are an overactive thyroid is responsible. When only one eye protrudes, the main causes are hemorrhages, inflations, or tumors which must be quickly dealt with. Often the protrusions are subtle, and instruments must be used to carefully compare the two eyes.

Double Vision

If you have ever experienced double vision when you were tired, after taking medication, or after drinking too much, you know how disturbing it can be. Sudden double vision without any apparent cause is very frightening. Regardless of the cause, it indicates that the two eyes are not pointing in the same direction.

In the cases of fatigue or drugs (including alcohol), there is interference with the brain's ability to control and coordinate the eye muscles. These are dealt with during the routine examination. A more serious matter is double vision which occurs suddenly and is present at all times. The probable cause is a small stroke, hemorrhage, or brain tumor. In most instances, proper treatment will gradually restore normal vision. Meanwhile, as a temporary aid, we will make special glasses to keep the double vision under control.

The Field of Vision

Normal vision is made up of two parts—accurate, sharp sight when looking directly at an object, coupled with a general awareness of the scene around you. To get the idea, do this experiment: Look straight ahead, hold your arms out at shoulder level and wiggle your fingers. With good peripheral vision, you should be aware of the movement of your fingers. (This also points out that at the extreme edges of your field of vision, the main attention-getter is motion.)

If you lose either the central vision or the peripheral vision, you can be considered legally blind. Clear, central vision is not enough by itself. Roll two sheets of paper into small tubes and look through them. You can watch TV and read, but try walking around in unfamiliar surroundings, or down a stairway. Driving a car would be impossible. Conversely, if your central vision is lost, you can walk around, but you cannot read or recognize faces well.

There are many diseases which can rob us of either the central or peripheral vision. Glaucoma is an example of one that gradually shrinks the peripheral vision until, in the final stage, it's like looking through the two paper tubes.

It is also possible for a small portion or section of the overall field to be lost in one eye. Usually, you will not be aware of the loss because the blank area is filled in by the sight from the other eye. If the loss is to the outside or downward, and cannot be filled in, you would probably find yourself frequently bumping into things.

By testing with small lights or colored spots moving across the entire normal field of vision, such blind spots or field losses can be located.

Aniseikonia

Aniseikonia means that there are unequal sized or shaped images sent to the brain from each eye. For normal, comfortable, binocular vision, the difference cannot be more than three or four percent. A greater amount can produce symptoms of mild to severe headaches and even double vision. Some people with this condition learned early in life to supress the image from one eye and thus avoid suffering. Perhaps they are the lucky ones, even though they only have the use of one eye.

We don't know how many people in this country suffer from the discomforts of aniseikonia, but our guess is that there may be millions. When the prescription for lenses in the two eyes differs drastically from lens to lens, aniseikonia is a probability. Sometimes the very glasses which correct other vision defects will produce the condition. That being the case, you would expect that all patients with tell-tale symptoms would be tested for aniseikonia. Unfortunately, very few doctors ever do. The reason is two-fold—instruments for proper testing are not readily available, and, correcting the condition is difficult and time consuming.

Since the symptoms can be relieved with special glasses or contact lenses, it should be done more often. It is our hope that in the next few years steps will be taken to manufacture reliable instruments to test for aniseikonia, and that doctors will make use of them.

Part IV

ALL ABOUT GLASSES
AND CONTACT LENSES

CHAPTER 14

HOW DO GLASSES WORK?

You were probably not too thrilled the first time you were told you needed glasses, but, as long as you must wear them, why not learn how they work?

Obviously, glasses are made up of lenses and a frame. The frame can be made of plastic, metal, or a combination of the two; its function is to keep the lenses positioned in front of your eyes. The part that sits on the bridge of your nose is called, quite logically, the "bridge," and the handles which fit on your ears are called "temples." Within certain limitations which will be described in later chapters, you can have free reign in your choice of frame styles and colors. It's the lenses, of course, which make the whole contraption so useful.

Basically, what is a lens? It doesn't have to be made out of glass or plastic to do its job. The only requirement is that it be transparent and capable of bending—refracting—light rays in a predetermined way. You could, if you put your mind to it, make a lens out of ice or gelatin and fulfill the basic requirement. It would make an interesting science fair project, but pretty strange glasses. No, we need something more durable.

Whether glass or plastic is used, it must be manufactured totally free of tiny air bubbles, striations and distortions; it requires very exacting techniques. There are plenty of rejects and "seconds" in lenses which, unfortunately, find their way to unscrupulous operators and so-called "bargain" houses.

The lens power is measured in units called diopters which are based on the extent to which the light rays passing through the lens will be bent. As the power of the lens increases, so does the thickness. Three types of lenses are commonly used to correct vision problems—convex, concave, and cylindrical.

The *convex* lens is thicker in the center than at the edges, and gathers light rays together towards a point. Remember when you were a kid and used a magnifying lens to focus the sun's rays on a piece of paper in order to start it burning? That was a convex lens. It is used in glasses for the farsighted eye which cannot bend the light rays as much as they should. If the eye is 2 diopters farsighted, a 2 diopter convex lens will compensate for it. It is also commonly used in reading glasses.

The *concave* lens is thinner at the center than at the edges, and spreads light rays apart. You could not use this lens to focus the sun's rays, because it never forms a real image anywhere. (The explanation involves physics—just take our word for it.) By putting this lens in front of the nearsighted eye, we can reduce the overall power to put the image neatly on the retina. A 1 diopter concave lens will correct 1 diopter of nearsightedness.

The *cylindrical* lens is shaped like a section of an auto tire, curved more in one direction than the other. It's very difficult to ascertain the direction of the curve by simply looking at your glasses. Sometimes you can recognize it this way: Hold the glasses about twenty inches in front of you and sight a straight line or edge through the lens. Slowly rotate the glasses clockwise and then counterclockwise. If the line tilts with or against the rotation of the glasses, it's a cylindrical lens and you have astigmatism. This type of lens must be carefully aligned in front of the eyes with an exact up and down orientation. Most often a cylindrical lens will be part of the prescription with a convex or concave lens.

Would you like to learn how to read a prescription for eyeglasses? A convex lens (for the farsighted eye) is written with a plus (+) symbol. A concave lens (for the nearsighted eye) is written with a minus (-) sign. If the prescription calls

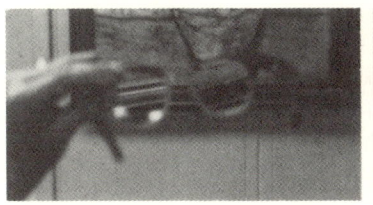

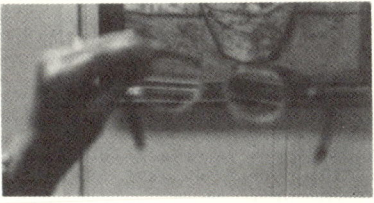

Rocking glasses back and forth to detect a cylinder lens which corrects astigmatism. The right lens has double the cylinder power and causes greater tilt of the lines.

for a +2.00, it's a 2 diopter lens for a farsighted eye, or it could be a 2 diopter reading lens for a presbyopic eye. A -2.50 is a 2½ diopter lens for a nearsighted eye. The higher the number, the stronger the lens.

For an eye with astigmatism the prescription might look like this:

-2.50   -1.00 axis 45

This is 2½ diopters of nearsightedness with 1 diopter of astigmatism. The axis indicates the orientation of the cylindrical part of the lens. It's based on the degrees of a protractor—180 is the horizontal, 90 the vertical meridians. The axis can be anywhere from 1 to 180.

A bifocal prescription will have additional numbers to indicate the strength of the reading part of the lens.

+1.75   -0.25 axis 95
add   +1.50

This is 1¾ diopters of farsightedness with ¼ diopter of astigmatism and an additional 1½ diopters of power for reading.

Sometimes a prism effect has to be incorporated into the prescription to deviate the light rays in a desired way.

-3.25   -0.75 axis 70   2$^\triangle$ IN

The little triangular figure designates a prism and in this case the direction of the base is inward, though it could be out, up or down.

You need one more piece of information in order to read your Rx—knowing which numbers are for which eye. The right eye is designated O.D. for the Latin *oculus dexter*; the left eye is O.S. for *oculus sinister*. O.U. is *oculus uterque*, both eyes.

You may still not be thrilled about having to wear glasses, but at least you now know what you're wearing.

CHAPTER 15

GETTING USED TO YOUR GLASSES

When you get glasses for the first time, or when there is a change in your prescription, it will upset your visual world. Certainly you can expect clearer sight and more comfortable vision, but along with that you will notice some strange side effects. Objects may look larger or smaller, closer or farther, and shapes may be distorted. Don't hit the panic button. These effects are only temporary and within a few days you should be unaware of them. But, why the problem in the first place? There are several reasons.

Because of technical limitations, only the very center of the lens has the exact prescription your eye needs. When you look away from the center (and you do every time you move your eyes), you're actually looking through a slightly different prescription. This difference increases towards the edge of the lens and causes shape and vision distortions. The thicker the lens the greater the distortions.

Two recent events have aggravated this general situation. First, federal law requires all lenses to be made shatter resistant. It's safer for you, but such lenses have to be thicker. Second, the very large glasses so popular now, mean *still thicker* lenses. In low power prescriptions, the distortions are manageable and you can adjust quickly. With high powers, the adjustment can be very difficult. *Large lenses should be avoided.*

Another factor influencing your sight with glasses, is the curvature of the lens. It is possible to grind lenses of the same power, but with a variety of curvatures. The lens can be made flat, or bulging like a bowl. So what? The curvature effects the image size seen through the lens. For example, a concave lens for a nearsighted person will produce a larger image with a deeper curve. If the prescription for your two eyes is quite different, the curvatures must be carefully controlled.

Has it ever happened to you that two supposedly identical pairs of glasses don't feel the same? It may be that they were not made with lenses of the same curvature.

If you are nearsighted and put glasses on for the first time, the world will look clearer, but smaller. Since the brain uses size as a judgment of distance (smaller objects are farther away), you will tend to think you are farther from things than you really are. You may spill a cup of coffee when you reach for it, because it's closer than you realize.

If you are farsighted, the opposite will happen. Objects will look clearer, but larger. So, you will judge things to be closer. You may reach for a doorknob and come up short. Over the span of a few days, you will regain your distance judgment.

These annoyances are minor compared to a first-time correction for astigmatism. Objects will be tilted and curved; your entire perspective will be in shambles. But, take heart. As confusing as things may be, they will slowly reassemble into a "normal" looking world within a few days.

A seemingly minor matter such as the distance between the lens and your eye will effect the power and image size. If you are farsighted and the glasses slip down your nose, the effective power and image size are increased. If you are nearsighted and wear your glasses at the end of your nose, the effective power and image size are reduced. The exact amount will vary with the length of your nose and the strength of the prescription.

All the annoying symptoms are intensified with high powers. The very nearsighted person also has to contend with unsightly, reflectively thick edges on the lenses. There are some ways to minimize this thickness, though they are all compromises. One way would be to use a glass which has greater power to bend light rays. Such glass is usually made by adding lead (trace amounts) to the glass mixture. The lenses are indeed thinner, but, as you would expect with lead, they are heavier. They are also more brittle. So, you have to trade off thinner edges for heavier glasses. (A recent development is a thinner glass made without lead and not quite as heavy.) Sometimes the edges can be made less noticeable by tinting either the lenses or the edges of the lenses. Finally, by choosing a smaller frame with smaller lenses, the edges will be thinner.

Some people are bothered by reflections from the surfaces of the lenses. You should have little trouble learning to ignore them, but if necessary, the reflections can be eliminated by coating the surfaces.

With large frames, unless you have very wide-set eyes, your eyes would rarely be centered in the middle of the lens. Yet, to get the best vision, the centers of the lenses must be in front of your pupils. Therefore, the lenses must be offset to

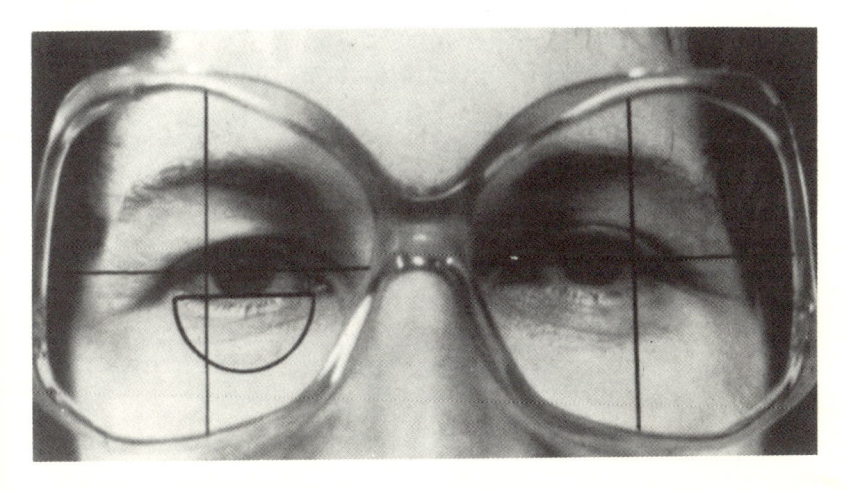

When a large frame is worn the eyes are not in the middle of the lens area. For comfortable seeing the optical center of the lenses must be positioned directly in front of the pupils. If a bifocal is required (as illustrated on the left) it must be offset nasally.

compensate for your actual eye position. If this is not done, it can upset your eye movements and focusing.

For all these reasons, it should be apparent to you that the making of glasses must not be a haphazard procedure. The measuring, fitting and aligning of the glasses has to be done accurately and knowledgeably. For your own good, the optometrist should oversee the entire process. If by chance the glasses have to be made elsewhere, you must bring them back to the optometrist for verification.

There are a number of things you should do to keep the glasses in good condition. When you put them on or take them off, use both hands and hold them by the temples. Try not to pull the temples outward. Because of various hair styles, women are especially guilty of this particular maneuver.

Never lay the glasses on a surface with the lenses down. Do this often enough, and you'll have scratches across the center of the lenses. Lay them on the temples or put them in the case.

Dirt can easily collect around the rims of the lenses. It's easy to remove with an old toothbrush and warm, soapy water.

If you have plastic lenses, always wash the dirt and grit off before wiping with a soft tissue or cloth. If you do not have immediate access to water, rather than wiping them when dry, just blow the dust off.

No matter how careful you are the glasses may become crooked and misaligned. You should return for proper frame adjustment to avoid discomfort and visual disturbances. The original fee for the glasses generally includes this service.

CHAPTER 16

BIFOCALS AND MULTIFOCALS

When the doctor told you that you needed bifocals, you may have protested, saying you were not that old. Actually, you probably weren't, even though a few grey hairs may have been showing up here and there. The average person begins to need bifocals in his or her 40's, and then only if he or she does reading or close work. Five hundred years ago when most people were illiterate and/or occupied with farming and tending chickens, bifocals were not necessary. Today, they are almost indispensable.

A simple way to describe a bifocal is to say that it has two prescriptions combined into one lens. A trifocal has three prescriptions combined into one lens.

That old kite flyer, Benjamin Franklin, came up with the idea for the bifocal in the 18th century. He found it very bothersome to switch from his distance glasses to his reading glasses and back again, all day long. His clever solution was to cut each set of lenses into half moons (lenses were round in those days), and put them together in one frame. The top half was his distance prescription and the bottom half his reading lenses.

No matter what form or shape modern bifocals have, they are essentially two pairs of glasses put together. As in Franklin's case, the most common reason for bifocals is presbyopia—when the eyes can no longer easily focus at near small objects. Prescribing reading glasses would cause distance vision to be blurred and you would have to take them off to see far away. If you also need glasses for distance seeing, then you are in Franklin's predicament. By placing the near prescription in only one part of the lens, there is no interference with normal distance seeing.

There are many variations in design of the modern bifocal lens. The particular one made for you must depend on your prescription, occupation, life style, etc. The reading segment can be any size, from very small to very large; its top edge can be flat, round or oval; it can be placed high or low in the lens. The possible combinations can run into the hundreds.

What are some of the factors in choosing a bifocal? How you use them is the main consideration. Take a symphony musician, for example, who must read the music at twenty-four inches, and also occasionally glance at the conductor thirty feet away. The musician needs a bifocal with a large reading area as well as a small portion at the top for distance seeing. At the other extreme is a golfer who needs clear distance vision, but also wants to see the score card. A tiny reading segment would be the choice. Not only must it be tiny, but it must be placed low in the lens so that it doesn't get into the line of sight when the golfer approaches the ball.

Each patient must have bifocals custom designed for his or her particular use. Many times it's impossible to design an "all purpose" bifocal for all activities. This becomes quite obvious when you consider that the musician could also be the golfer. He or she should not expect to use the same bifocal for both activities, any more than he or she should wear evening clothes on the golf course.

The prescription strength of the reading portion can be made (within reason) for the distance at which you will use it. A carpenter working at arm's length wants to see clearly at about twenty-four inches. A woman who uses a sewing machine and makes her own clothes, would prefer to see clearly at about fifteen inches. That doesn't mean you have to be exactly twenty-four inches or fifteen inches away in these cases. Depending on your age, there is a leeway of clear vision, both closer and behind these distances.

Certain occupations require rather unusual lenses. Here's an interesting one. We can put two reading segments into the lens, one at the bottom and one at the top. This is suitable for a druggist who must read labels on shelves well above eye level. An electrician doing overhead wiring would also find this type of lens useful.

Trifocals are three pairs of glasses in one. Why would anyone need three different prescriptions? As you get older and the eye's focusing flexibility gets weaker, you may not be able to see clearly at all distances with a bifocal. The distance prescription at the top of the lens will let you see clearly from about five feet, all the way out to the stars; the reading segment will let you read up close. This leaves an area from about one and one-half feet to four feet which will be blurry. If you need or want clear vision at that distance, the in-between segment of the trifocal will supply it. A typical example might be a person who cheats at cards and has trouble seeing the secret markings across the table.

In regular bifocals or trifocals, there is an abrupt change in the prescription from one section to the next. One type of lens has a continuously changing prescription from the distance to the reading power. Theoretically, all seeing would be clear if you were to look through the appropriate part of the lens. In practice, some people find it a marvelous advantage, while others can't seem to cope with the constantly changing focus and distortions. These multifocals can be called "invisible" because there is no noticeable dividing line between the sections. One manufacturer makes an invisible bifocal which may be more cosmetically acceptable to some people, but this bifocal suffers from bad vision distortions.

When you get your first bifocals, you'll have to develop new seeing habits. New patterns must be established in head and eye movement relationships. For one thing, when walking down stairs, don't just lower your eyes. If you do, you will be looking through the reading segment which is meant to be used at less than two feet. Unless you are

Bifocals and Multifocals: Some of the many styles of bifocals and trifocals drawn to illustrate the variety of designs.

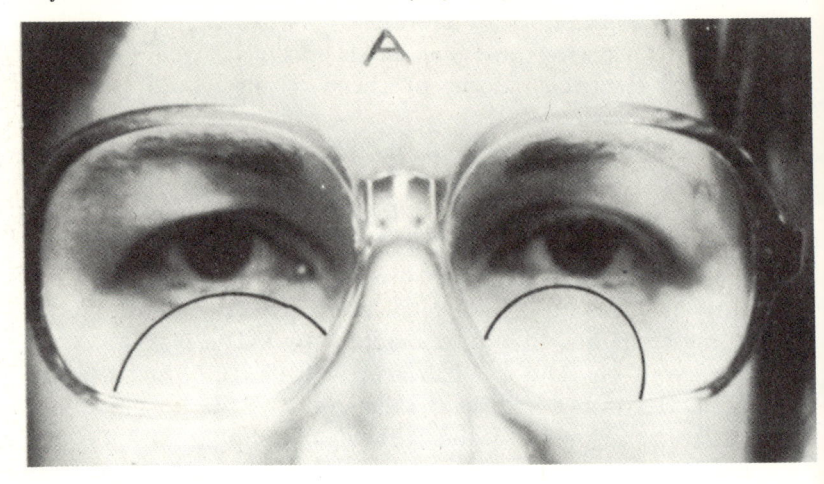

Two types of round top bifocals.

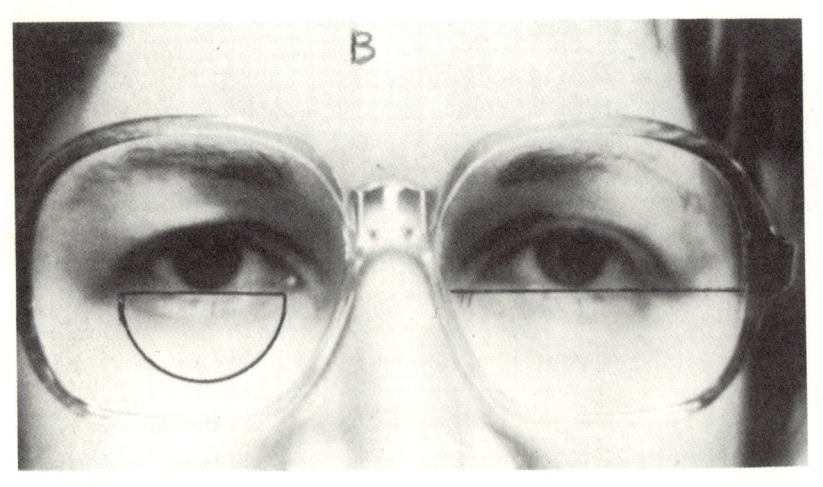

On the left is a flat top bifocal. On the right is an executive bifocal.

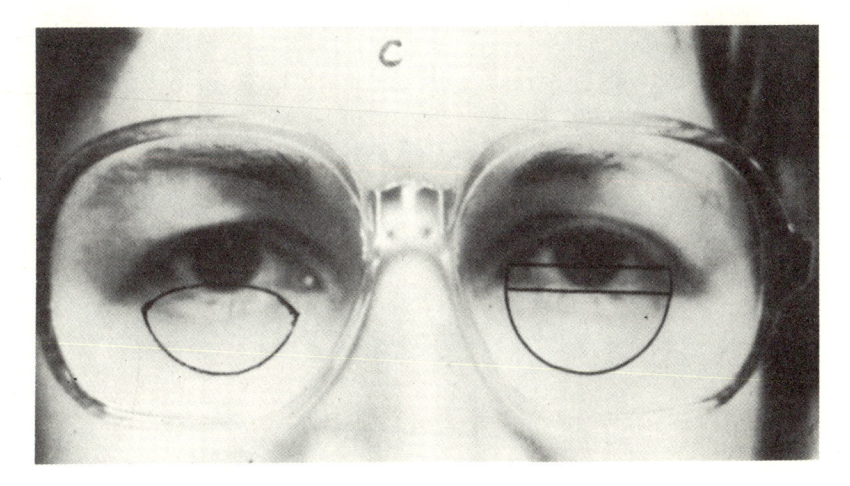

On the left is an oval top bifocal. On the right is a flat top trifocal.

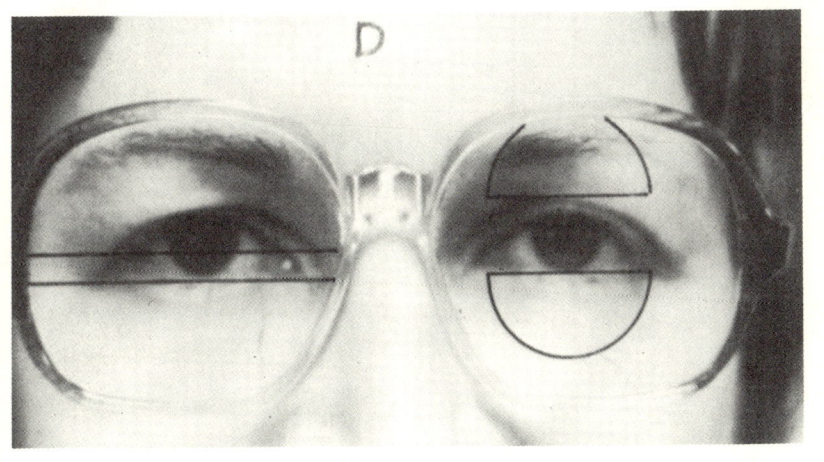

On the left is an executive trifocal. On the right is a dual bifocal.

extremely short, the stairs are farther away than two feet. To see the stairs clearly, lower your chin to your chest and sight through the upper part of the lenses.

Another common problem for beginning bifocal wearers is their attempt to read a notice on a bulletin board. Simply raise your chin so that the reading segment is brought into position.

Most people learn to use bifocals fairly rapidly, and within a week or ten days have everything mastered. A few people just never seem to be able to get the hang of it and must use two pairs of glasses. If you are one of these people, have the optometrist reassess your vision needs. You may have been trying to use the wrong bifocal for your particular needs.

CHAPTER 17

SUNGLASSES AND TINTED LENSES

Sunglasses are, of course, a type of tinted lenses. Because of their widespread and common use, we have given them top billing. You probably use sunglasses for protection from the intense glare of sunlight, but do you know what you are actually protecting yourself from? The light which our eyes use to see is only a tiny fraction of the radiation given off by the sun. You physics buffs know that the radiation extends from the miniscule gamma rays through X-rays, ultra-violet, visible light, infra-red, and on, to the very long radio waves. It is no coincidence that the visible light we see is precisely that radiation which is reflected from solid objects such as trees, rocks, and people.

If you have ever idly wished that you had X-ray vision, you would quickly change your mind the first time you walked into a brick wall which is transparent to X-rays. Note how many people are injured walking into glass doors which are transparent to visible light. Obviously, our visual system evolved to give us the most useful information about our surroundings.

Some of the radiation from the sun (or artificial sources) is harmful. But, to be harmful or have any effect at all, the radiation must be absorbed. No absorption, no effect. For example, radio waves pass through our bodies without being absorbed and without any effect. On the other hand, X-rays are absorbed, are dangerous, and must be shielded with lead (which absorbs them).

The two types of radiation we are normally subjected to

and which may cause eye problems, are the ultra-violet and the infra-red from sunlight. Although you can sense infra-red as heat on your skin, both of these are invisible to our eyes. The ultra-violet cannot be sensed, but its absorption by the skin leads to a suntan or sunburn.

Let's see what these rays can do to your eye. The ultra-violet is almost totally absorbed by the cornea, the balance by the lens inside the eye. Therefore, because of the absorption, any dire effects will be mainly on the cornea. The surface layer of the cornea can blister and hurt much more than any sunburn you've ever had. This sometimes happens to people who read under a sunlamp, not realizing that the ultra-violet is reflected off the paper onto the eye. It is a very painful experience. Only the short-wave ultra-violet rays are harmful. The long-wave ultra-violet used commonly as "black lights" to make fluorescent paints glow, are harmless. This should be good news to the men who have been watching Go-Go dancers by the pulsating flashes of strobe "black lights." And, to the Go-Go dancers as well.

The infra-red (heat) rays are absorbed partly by the cornea, partly by the lens, but a good portion gets through to the retina. There is evidence that infra-red rays are a factor in causing burns on the retina. That's exactly what can happen when you look at the sun's corona during an eclipse. While the intensely bright visible glare is blocked, massive amounts of infra-red can enter the eye and focus on the retina. Depending on the duration and intensity, the retina may be burned, causing permanent scars and loss of vision.

By now you get the idea that sunglasses must not only cut down on visible glare, but must definitely filter out ultra-violet and infra-red.

If you have sunglasses and think you are protected, we have a surprise for you. There is *no way* for you to tell by either the color or the darkness whether they actually filter out the harmful rays. The color of the lens is not what counts. Absorption of harmful rays depends on the chemical ingredient added to the glass to produce the color. A dark green glass made properly, will absorb all the harmful rays, but another green glass made without the proper ingredients will not. Worse than that, because the imitation lenses reduce the visible glare (nature's warning signal), it actually may be more harmful than wearing no colored lenses. (It's like the eclipse situation we described before. The glare is blocked while the infra-red gets through to your eyes.)

The confusion in the field of ready-made sunglasses is deplorable. You can find glasses with every conceivable color and degree of darkness promoted as sunglasses. Some are made with glass lenses and some with plastic lenses. Those which contain *ground* and *polished* dark *glass* lenses offer good protection from intense sunlight. Those which contain *molded* glass lenses are optically poor, full of distortions and aberrations. Can you tell the good from the bad by the labelling? Incredibly, no! For some reason, the logic of which escapes us, the excellent sunglasses manufactured by several reputable firms, contain no written clue to their quality or absorption characteristics. They are merely labelled as shatter-resistant which is required of even the worst junk.

If they contain plastic lenses (and most of them do), you can be sure of one thing—they do NOT filter out the infra-red radiation. The nature of the plastic material is such that it *does* filter out ultra-violet, but virtually *none* of the infra-red. You may be looking cool, but you may be simultaneously "cooking" your eye. (Recently, a plastic sunglass lens capable of filtering infra-red has been made available to the profession. Your chances of finding it on the racks of a supermarket or drugstore are less than finding a pearl in an oyster at your local eatery.)

In our view, there should be federal standards for all sunglasses. The public is at the mercy of anyone who decides to make colored lenses and call them sunglasses. Until there are standards, we suggest that before you buy, ask if they filter out ultra-violet and infra-red. A dumb-look response is your signal to go elsewhere. (If you're looking for good sunglasses, don't expect to find them in a grocery store,

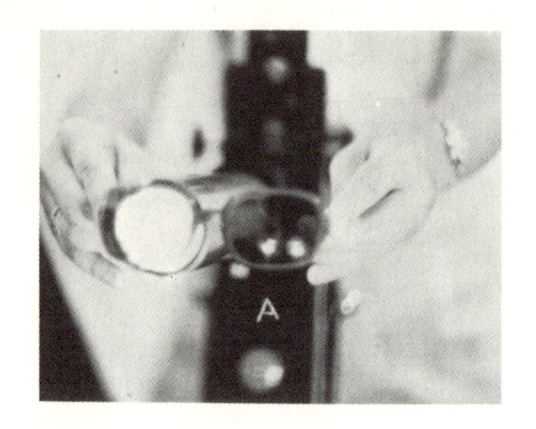

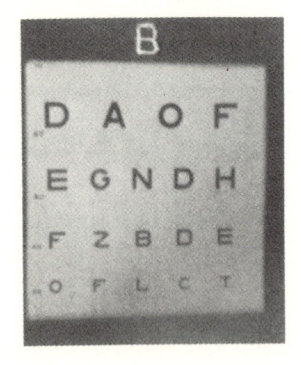

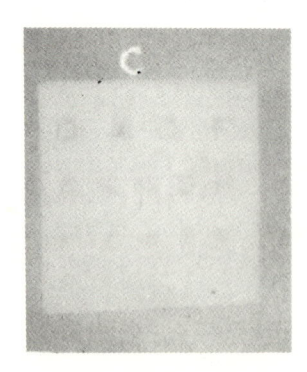

To check neutrality of lenses we hold "sunglasses" in front of projection tube. Photo B shows clear letters through good lenses. Photo C shows blurred image which results from distortion in lenses.

variety store, gas station, cigar counter, etc.)

Which brings us to the latest fad for wearing cosmetic tints or "fun" glasses, as they are called. Whether they are ready-made or made up in your prescription, the colors are much too light to be taken seriously as sunglasses. We suppose there is no real harm for younger people wearing them if they think it will put more "fun" in their lives. But, they must understand that their eyes are not being protected from sunlight. For older people, however, these tinted lenses are ill-advised since they may cause a reduction in sight both indoors and at night. You oldsters will have to find some other way to have "fun."

The newest wrinkles in this fad are the gradient tinted lenses which are dark on top and light on the bottom. They were originally developed for pilots who must cope with a bright outside sky, yet be able to read the dim cockpit dials. It's a clever solution for this situation. But, for the average person, there is usually just as much harmful glare bouncing up from sidewalks, beaches, or water, to make the light bottoms of these lenses useless for protection.

The best all-around sunglasses contain properly made *dark grey glass* lenses. The "smoke" tint permits you to see colors in an almost normal way. Next in line are good green glass lenses followed by the browns. Blue and yellow, regardless of how dark, are no good for sunglasses. Yellow lenses can be used by hunters, pilots, tennis players, etc., to increase visibility on a cloudy or hazy day. They are effective for this purpose, but only this purpose.

Good sunglasses are not cheap. But, don't be misled into getting an expensive pair strictly on the advertising endorsement of some celebrity. Chances are this person doesn't know infra-red from a hole in the ground.

Plastic polarized sunglasses are touted for reducing glare coming off flat reflecting surfaces such as water, but they suffer from the same lack of infra-red filtering as any plastic lenses. If you can get *glass* polarized lenses, then you've really got something good (and expensive). In generally cool

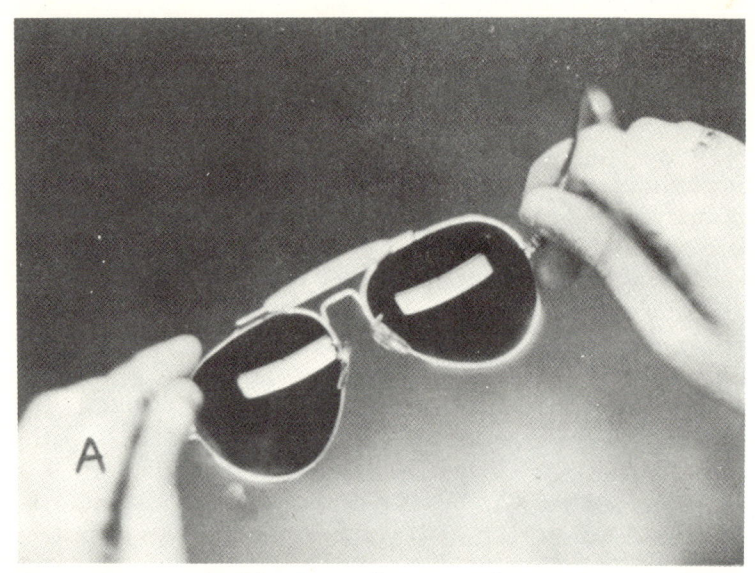

Good sunglasses should reflect a fluorescent fixture crisply and cleanly as in A. Photo B shows poor, distorted reflection from bad "sunglasses."

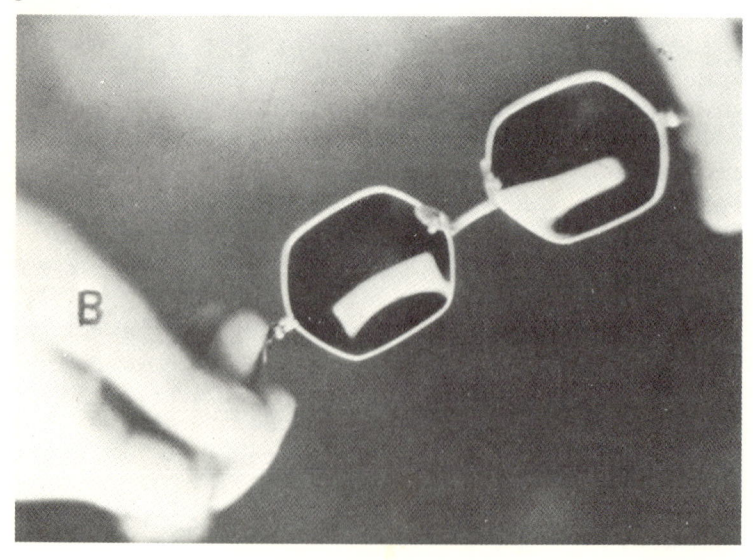

climates, good plastic sunglasses may be sufficient for you. In hot climates or in areas with hot summers they are inadequate.

There are two ways to make prescription sunglasses. (1) The glass itself is colored before the Rx is ground into it. (2) The finished clear lens is chemically coated to whatever hue desired. The latter method has the advantage of being evenly tinted regardless of the lens thickness. An extra attraction is the capability to remove the coating at any time or to change to a different color. This vacuum-coating method is also used to deposit an anti-reflective layer on the lens surfaces to reduce the internal reflections. You have probably seen camera lenses and binoculars with this faint blueish-toned coating.

About ten years ago, one glass manufacturer developed a photochromic glass which has the ability to darken when exposed to ultra-violet, and lighten when the ultra-violet is absent. The public has been bombarded with advertising for these "automatic sunglasses." Our evaluation of this implied claim is, "Bunk!" The range of these lenses is not sufficient to go from completely clear to completely dark. After repeated exposures to ultra-violet, the lenses will retain a smokey-pink hue even at night. This puts them into the same category as "fun" glasses. The admonition to older people against wearing "fun glasses," applies to the photochromic lenses as well. (In our opinion, too many photochromic bifocals are being prescribed. Very few people benefit enough to overcome the drawbacks of reduced sight and lessened reading ability in low light.)

Another problem with photochromic glasses is that the lenses do not darken enough to protect the eyes from glare such as might be encountered at a beach. This would result in retinal cell "bleaching" and degraded night vision. In other words, if you spent the day at the seaside, your drive home on darkened roads could be hazardous. Naturally, this also applies to pale sunglasses, no sunglasses, "fun" glasses, and gradient density lenses.

One peculiarity of the photochromic glass is that it darkens more in cold weather than in hot weather, making it more suitable for skiing than for beach hopping. Finally, since these lenses do *not* filter out infra-red, they cannot be considered as true sunglasses for warm climate use.

Now, let's briefly examine other needs for tinted lenses besides sunlight. One large area is in various industrial processes which involve spill-overs of ultra-violet and infra-red. Steelmaking, welding and glassblowing are typical examples. If you have ever watched a glassblower making those intricate figurines, you may have noticed that he or she was wearing tinted lenses for protection against the intense infra-red of the hot flame. The people in industry are generally well aware of these potential hazards, and every effort is made to protect the workers with the proper tinted lenses.

The problem of glare from visible light is not only related to brightness. You can have very annoying glare in low illumination. The most common example is watching television in a totally dark room. The sharp contrast is quite fatiguing; we suggest that you have a background light on in the room.

Artificial light reflecting off white paper, desk tops and other shiny surfaces can also be irritants, and are frequent complaints of office personnel. Sometimes when we examine individuals with this complaint, we find a visual problem of which they were unaware. Correcting the visual problem will often eliminate what was thought to be a sensitivity to light. Otherwise, lightly tinted lenses may be prescribed.

There are several eye diseases which can increase a person's sensitivity to light. A sudden change in tolerance to light calls for an eye examination. With any kind of corneal injury, it will be almost impossible to keep the eyes open even in normal illumination. Dark lenses are quite useful while the healing process is going on. On a lesser note, large, dark sunglasses are also useful in hiding a blackened eye, no matter how it was obtained.

SELECTION GUIDE TO TINTED-GLASS LENSES

PERCENTAGE OF ABSORPTION

Color		Ultra Violet	Visible Light	Infra Red	Uses
CLEAR		7%	7%	7%	
PINK	Light	95%	10%	10%	Cuts glare from
	Medium	95%	15-20%	10%	artificial lights.
	Dark	95%	45-50%	15%	
BLUE	Light	95%	10%	5%	Cuts glare from
	Medium	95%	25%	10%	artifical lights.
	Dark	95%	70%	12%	Cosmetic. NOT for sun.
GREEN	Light	75%	15%	55%	Cataract glasses.
	Medium	99%	35%	98%	Cool climate sunglasses.
	Dark	99%	70%	99%	Good sunglasses.
BROWN	Light	95%	20-40%	35%	Cool climate sunglasses
	Medium	97%	65%	50%	and cuts through blue haze.
	Dark	99%	80%	80%	Sunglasses.
GRAY	Light	95%	20-40%	60%	Cool climate sunglasses or
	Medium	97%	60%	70%	not too sensitive to light.
	Dark	98%	80%	80%	Best all-around sunglasses.
YELLOW		95%	15%	10%	Increase visibility in haze and fog.
PHOTO-	Light	85%	15-20%	15%	General wear and winter
CHROMIC	Dark	85%	20-70%	15%	sports. Sunglasses in cool climate.

These figures are averages and may vary from manufacturer to manufacturer. The exact thickness of the lens may also be a factor in the absorption.

Any tinted lens should only be worn at the appropriate time. Sunglasses whould not be worn at night or in dim illumination. Never, never wear sunglasses while driving at night. While it may reduce the glare from oncoming headlights, it will also reduce your ability to see. On a dark night, it has been estimated that sunglasses will reduce your seeing distance by one third. Traveling at 55 miles per hour, can you afford the luxury of one-third less reaction time?

CHAPTER 18

SHATTER-RESISTANT GLASS OR PLASTIC LENSES

Several years ago, a TV commercial for a well-known retail optical house showed a child throwing a rock at another child. The recipient of this unwanted gift was wearing glasses; the rock bounced merrily off the "shatter proof" lenses without any harm. We wonder how many kids decided that this was great fun and started throwing rocks at those wearing glasses, with far different results. No glass is ever completely shatter proof or unbreakable, despite the commercial's clever but misleading wording.

Since January of 1972, federal law has required most lenses (there are a few exceptions) to be made shatter resistant. This means exactly what it says—resistant to shattering, not immune to shattering. They are neither safety lenses nor unbreakable, and should not be thought of that way. Of course, shatter-resistant lenses were in use for a long time before the law went into effect. They were prescribed regularly for kids, sports figures, and industry workers.

To be considered shatter resistant, the lens must be capable of withstanding the impact of a half ounce, five-eighths of an inch steel ball dropped onto the lens from a height of fifty inches. For industrial use, the lens must withstand a heavier steel ball drop. Ordinary glass subjected to this test would shatter into tiny sharp fragments and could cause serious eye injury.

There are several ways to make lenses shatter resistant. The most commonly employed method is by heat treating. The lens is heated and then quickly cooled by a blast of air. A newer method is to chemically harden the lens by keeping it in a super hot salt solution for twelve to fifteen hours. Finally, glass lenses can be made shatter resistant by laminating a thin sheet of plastic into the center like a slice of ham between slices of bread.

A drawback for the patient is that no matter which method is used, the lens must be thicker (a minimum of 2.2 mm for regular and 3 mm for industrial use) and consequently heavier. The thicker lenses are cosmetically disturbing and the added weight is uncomfortable on the nose.

Any scratches or pits that develop on the lens will seriously compromise its resistance to breakage. We have had an occasional patient return with lenses that apparently shattered without being struck. Perhaps the lenses were scratched, but since we're not sure, we call it a "spontaneous breakage." Apparently, the shatter-resistant glass lens is not the ultimate solution.

Enter the plastic lens. The word "plastic" tends to evoke thoughts of the many plastic products which are cheaply made and short lived. There is a great difference between those plastics and the new plastic lenses.

First of all, the material used to make these lenses is optically just as good, and four times as impact resistant as hardened glass. Even if a strong enough blow causes breakage, the pieces are not sharp and have little penetrating force. Not only is the lens quite safe, but it has the amazing ability to shed sparks from welding and grinding which would pit glass lenses. A couple of nice side benefits—it is half the weight of glass and doesn't fog up as readily. With all these advantages you would suppose that everyone should wear plastic lenses. Not so, because for some patients there are a few disadvantages.

The main disadvantage is that the surface is not quite as hard as glass. This means that the plastic lenses are a little more susceptible to getting scratched, and better care is

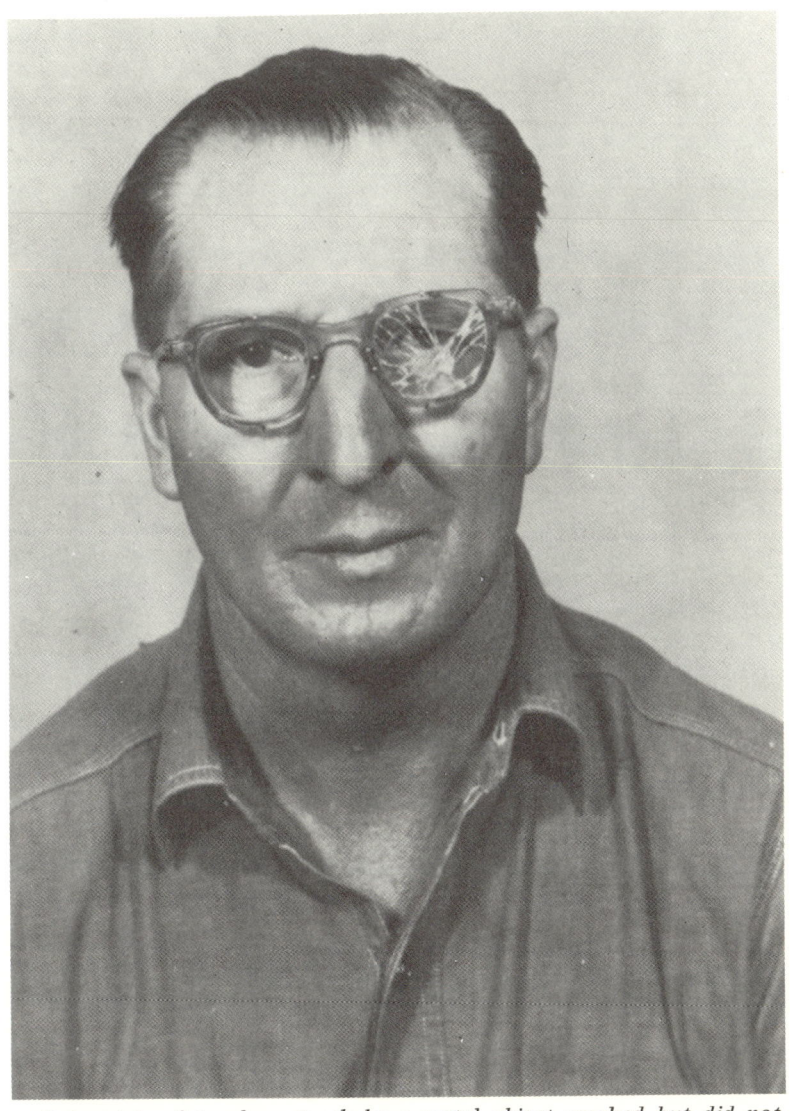

Industrial safety glass struck by a metal object cracked but did not shatter. Photo courtesy of Illinois Society for the Prevention of Blindness.

required, although it is possible to treat the surfaces for increased scratch resistance. For a comparable prescription, the plastic lens is slightly thicker than glass, but still much lighter. This is a problem only in a very strong nearsighted correction. If you're getting sunglasses, the plastic lenses are not as effective in warm climates; they do not filter out any of the infra-red radiation. Lastly, they are a bit more expensive than glass lenses.

Please do weigh the pros and cons to find out which lens material is best for you. For a rough and tumble boy or girl who will not properly handle the plastic lenses, glass will take longer to get scratched up. For a welder, the plastic lenses will far outlast the glass. If you're involved in active sports, you will like the lightness of the plastic, plus the fact that it doesn't fog up when you perspire. As a rule of thumb, in most types of corrections, adults can be more comfortable with the plastic lenses.

CHAPTER 19

WHAT CONTACT LENSES ARE AND HOW THEY WORK

There are two questions uppermost in the mind of anyone thinking about contact lenses: "Can I wear them?" and "Will they hurt?" The second question is easier to answer. You've had the experience of a tiny piece of dust irritating the eye, and by extension you expect a contact lens, which is so much bigger, to hurt like the devil. But, the cornea (the clear cover of the eye where the contact fits) is very choosy in its pain sensitivity. It is violently responsive to tiny things touching it, but NOT sensitive to larger objects. It seems odd until you realize that a large object touches your cornea all the time—your lids. Yet, you feel no pain each time you blink. A contact lens, which is large compared to a speck of dust, won't hurt either, provided it's properly fitted.

We're not implying that you won't feel a thing the first time you put a hard contact lens on your eye. You will feel some discomfort, mostly the inside of your lid rubbing across the edge of the lens at each blink. Getting used to this lid sensation is part of getting used to contacts. (This problem is eliminated, however, with the soft lenses.) The essential adaptation which determines whether you can wear contacts, requires the cornea to alter the way it obtains oxygen and nutrients. Whether you can wear them then, depends on your motivation, the skill of the doctor, your eyes, and your prescription. If this seems to duck the question, let's simply say that most people who really want to, can.

In the past dozen years there has been an explosive increase in the use of contact lenses. There are several million people wearing them, and, we wouldn't be surprised if there were an equal number of people who bought the lenses and stuffed them into a drawer. There are many reasons for these "failures," the chief one being the poor fitting techniques done by incompetent people.

The lure of a fast buck attracted thousands of semi-professionals into the contact lens field. You will find their ads in print, on TV and in the yellow pages. Their ads are generally better than their fitting techniques. As a good rule of thumb, don't entrust your eyes to anyone who has to advertise. Beware of any "sales" or "bargains" in contacts; avoid anyone who thinks so little of your eyes and vision.

In the 1970s, the introduction of the flexible, soft lenses made it possible to fit many previously unsuccessful wearers. But, the soft lenses are not for everyone, anymore than the hard lenses are for everyone. In a later section we will discuss the pros and cons of the various lens designs.

Most people are amazed to learn that contact lenses have been around since the 19th century. Until some twenty years ago, with the introduction of the small corneal lenses, their use was very limited.

The early contact lenses were very large, fit over the entire eye, and were made of glass. Can you imagine the motivation for someone to put a fragile piece of glass on the eye? It was not a matter of vanity. They were worn by people who could only get good vision with contacts—glasses couldn't help them.

In the 1940s, the development of clear, transparent plastic which could be fashioned into contacts, eliminated the inherent danger of the glass lenses. They were still big and bulky, however, covering the cornea and the sclera (the white part of the eye). The introduction of a thin, small lens which rests on the cornea, held there by simple capillary attraction, was the breakthrough which made it possible for many more people to be fitted. What does that mean? The natural moisture of the cornea holds the lens in place. If you moisten your finger and touch it to a piece of paper you will notice how it clings.

Now that you've got the idea, we must point out that your finger is not like the cornea; nor is a piece of paper like a contact lens. The cornea is actually a very unique structure in many ways. Besides being transparent and selective in its pain reaction, it has no direct blood supply. Consequently, it must get its oxygen and nutrients needed by every living tissue, from the air and tear layer. If anything blocks the air or tear layer, the metabolism and transparency will suffer. The ultimate contact lens would permit air and fluids to pass through easily. We are not yet at that stage of the art, but undoubtedly it is somewhere in the future.

None of the F.D.A. approved lenses now in use allow either air or tears to pass through. So, how do you maintain the health of the cornea? That, of course, is the crucial factor in fitting a lens to the eye.

Let's take a closer, detailed look at the cornea. Under very high magnification, it turns out that the cornea is not really spherical. Careful measurements of the surface curvature, which must be taken during the initial examination, indicate that the center region peaks to a plateau while the edges near the side of the eye flatten out.

A contact lens must approximate this shape, but only approximate it. If we made a contact lens to match the curvature exactly, to fit like a glove, so to speak, it would be intolerable. A snug fit would prevent any tear exchange, and the cornea would quickly become swollen and cloudy. The lens has to be designed so that each blink causes some movement, which in turn causes a pumping action that exchanges stale for fresh tears.

If the lens is too loose, you'll get plenty of tear exchange, but the lens will slip around, rub and irritate the cornea, and may fall out. We need a delicate balance between snugness and looseness which is achieved by controlling the curvature, size, thickness, and edge bevels of the contact lens. When you realize that the lens may be only one-third an inch in diameter, with a thickness of perhaps one-hundredth of an inch, that's a lot to build into a tiny piece of plastic. But, it must be done if you are to wear contact lenses.

Before we both go through all this trouble, are there any advantages to contacts besides the very obvious cosmetic ones? Quite a few, really.

1. Vision is more natural and in almost true size. With glasses, things may look larger or smaller.
2. Since contacts move with the eyes when looking to the sides, there are no distortions such as you may experience with glasses.
3. Side vision is better because it's unobstructed by a frame.
4. When you're out in rain or snow, there is nothing to catch the drops and flakes.
5. Contacts can't steam up from temperature changes or perspiration.
6. If the lens correction for each eye is very different, as after a cataract operation, the use of contacts is the best way for the two eyes to work together.
7. Some people with tendencies for an eye to cross, have better eye movement control with contacts than with glasses.
8. Nearsighted individuals will find that less frequent changes are needed in their prescriptions.

As an offshoot of the last point, there is a branch of specialties called orthokeratology, which seeks to reduce and eliminate nearsightedness by changing contacts at regular intervals to alter the shape of the cornea. While some optometrists have obtained marked success with this procedure, many years of study and data are needed to confirm its safety and permanence. (For a fuller discussion see Chapter 31, Control of Nearsightedness.)

There are a few instances when contacts are the ONLY way to get good vision—when the cornea is scarred, has an irregular shape, or in keratoconous, a disease which causes the cornea to thin and bulge out.

Contact lenses are made of various types of plastic materials. The two basic types in use now are hard and water repellent, or soft and water absorbent. (Laboratories are working on many combinations such as soft and non-water absorbent; hard, but gas permeable, etc. We lack enough clinical information on these combinations to evaluate them at this time.)

The traditional hard lens used for the last quarter of a century, is quite rigid. Over the years, improved technology has produced very thin lenses which can be flexed between your fingers, but once on the eye are essentially firm.

The newer soft lenses can be folded and rolled in your hand and easily yield to the pressure of the lids. These lenses contain a percentage of moisture. When a soft contact is on your eye, it absorbs your own tears. The exact amount of absorption varies among manufacturers, from 20% to 80%.

Now, are you ready for contacts? Talk it over with your optometrist. If he or she doesn't fit them, you will be referred to someone who does. The fitting must be done personally by the doctor, and should not be sloughed off to an assistant. It's a good idea to ask the optometrist before you commit yourself. Don't let anyone else near your eyes. Also, find out if lens adjustments are done right in the office. You'll save a lot of time if the lenses don't have to be returned to the laboratory for every slight modification. Doing it in the office gives the doctor better control, and the benefits of the change can be verified much faster.

Being fitted with contact lenses demands your time, money, and perseverance. In return, the doctor's responsibility is to attend to you personally, including the very important follow-up care. Just handing you a prescription with the words "contact lenses" on it, is sheer nonsense. If the doctor is too busy or too lazy to take the time needed to fit the contact personally, get your eyes out of that office. There is always the strong possibility that this doctor just doesn't know how to do it.

What should you expect the doctor to do? First, a complete, regular examination. Something may show up which will rule out contacts or make them a poor choice. Then, specifically for contacts, he or she will measure the curvature of your cornea—the entire cornea, not just the center. In effect, the doctor has to plot out a topographical map of your cornea.

When the optometrist has this information, the two of you should discuss which lenses would be advisable, the hard or the soft. Perhaps you are lucky and your eyes are suitable for either type. In this case, after reading the next chapter, you will be able to make a decision.

Whichever are decided on, at this point, many doctors prefer to try a few diagnostic lenses on your eye. It affords a chance to evaluate the physical fit of the lenses before ordering a set for you.

There are many types of special hard lenses for unusual eyes and vision conditions. There are also bifocal and multifocal contacts made in several different modes. All of these special lenses require additional expertise by the doctor.

CHAPTER 20

HARD LENSES VS. SOFT

If you pressed us for a one-word summary of the advantage of the soft lens, that word would be "comfort." The patients who most appreciate this are former hard lens wearers, who stopped using them because of discomfort. When we put a soft lens on the eye, they are absolutely astounded by the lack of any annoying sensation. "I don't feel a thing!" is the common happy remark from anyone trying soft lenses on for the first time.

If, again, you pressed us for a one-word summary of the biggest drawback of the soft lenses, that word would be "sight" (with "cleaning" running a close second). For some people the sight is good, for some it is mediocre, and for some it is just plain bad.

The rigidity of the hard lens makes it excellent for vision. In fact, to correct corneal astigmatism (a sight defect caused by the cornea being a little "out of round"), you need only a hard contact lens on the eye. The lens' even round surface compensates for the cornea's uneven surface and eliminates the astigmatism. If you are also nearsighted or farsighted, the appropriate power is ground into the lens.

In sharp contrast, if you have a large amount of astigmatism, the soft lens is at a disadvantage. The lens tends to conform to the shape of the cornea, and if that surface shape is uneven, the contact's surface will also be uneven. For another thing, the softness of the lens allows it to buckle slightly when you blink or when you read. This can make the vision somewhat variable. Proper lens selection can keep this at a minimum, but your own judgment is important. If you think your vision just isn't crisp and clear enough with the best lens we can prescribe, then soft lenses are not for you.

If you do get good vision with the soft lenses, there are a flock of additional advantages you will enjoy. It's almost impossible for them to fall out of the eye by themselves—marvelous for sports. Dust and dirt can't get between the lens and the cornea to cause irritation. It takes fewer days to adapt to them, and even if you accidentally overwear them, there is little danger of injury or infection to the eye. You can freely interchange the wearing of glasses and soft contacts. Most people are less light sensitive with soft lenses, even though they are not available in tinted form. They are better for night driving because side glare or sparkle is hardly evident.

There is difficulty, however, in keeping them clean and uncontaminated with foreign matter. The lens is soft because it absorbs water or tears. But, it is very democratic and will absorb just about anything, including hair spray, perfume, deodorant, toxic gases, and, you name it. The first rule is to keep your eyes closed when there are mists in the air, a rule which might be tough to follow. Once the foreign material is absorbed by the lens, it may or may not come out with cleaning.

The most common contaminant we have seen in soft lenses is the secretion from your own lids. Try avoiding that! There are several glands in the lids which produce oily liquids to keep the eye moist. This fluid contains fats and proteins which must be scrupulously cleaned from the surface of the lenses before they are sterilized, or it will cause a gradual buildup. When enough has accumulated, the lenses become uncomfortable and the vision deteriorates.

After many years of testing and obtaining approval from the F.D.A., an enzymatic cleaner became available to remove the protein deposited on the lenses. Unless you get some non-protein material into the lens, by using this cleaner regularly, it will keep the contact lenses clear and comfortable.

Some other undesirable aspects of the soft lenses are a shorter material life, chance of ripping or tearing, and discoloration. If your vision changes and you require a different power, unlike the hard lenses, the prescription cannot be reground. Further, some people find them uncomfortable in dry climates or in certain industrial environments when there are fumes or mists in the air. A lack of humidity in the air such as might be encountered in an overheated home or office, might also make the soft lenses less comfortable. Finally, the soft lenses are more expensive than the hard contacts.

If your eyes lend themselves to a choice of either type, we would suggest you lean towards the soft lenses. The wearing ease and lack of irritation to the eyes tips the scale in their favor.

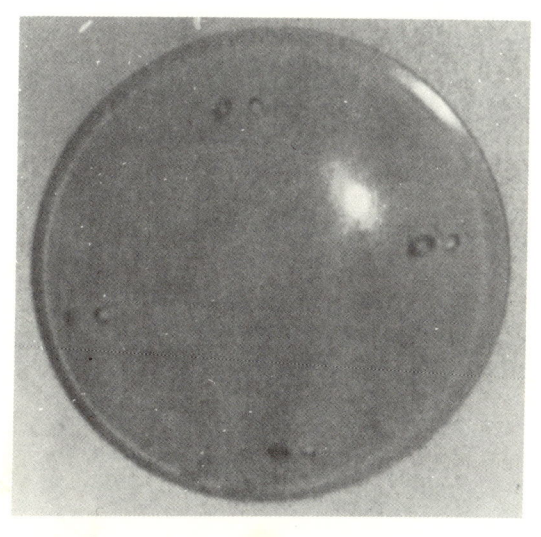

Tiny holes are sometimes used to increase tear circulation.

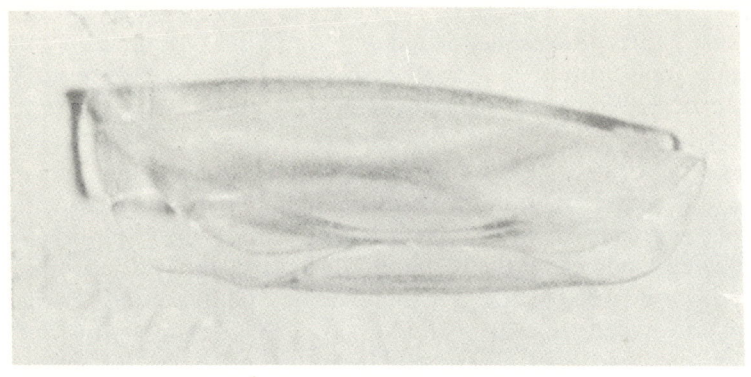

A dried and shriveled soft contact lens. Wetting will restore it to its normal shape.

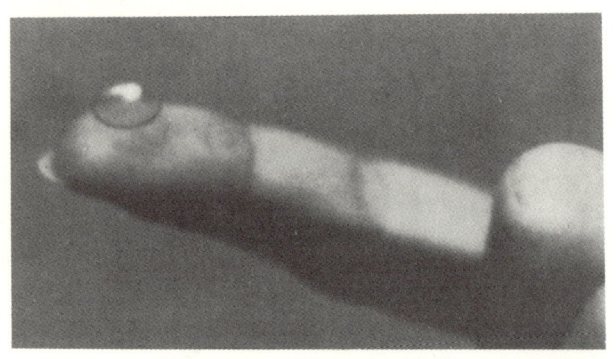

A typical hard contact lens.

A soft contact lens can be folded.

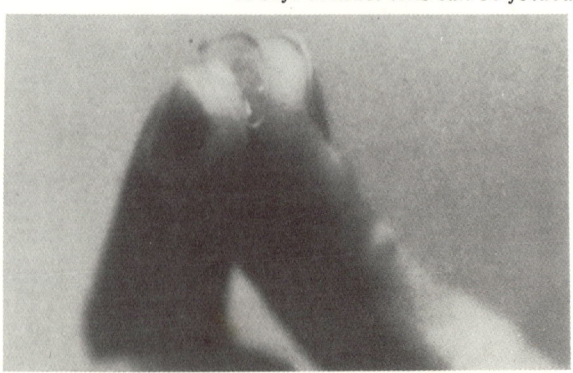

HARD VS. SOFT CONTACT LENS GUIDE

	HARD	SOFT
SIGHT	Generally excellent	Ranges from poor to excellent. Sometimes variable.
COMFORT	Discomfort at first. Mild sensations.	Virtually no sensation from start.
INJURY & INFECTIONS	Some chance.	Almost none.
LIGHT SENSITIVE	Mild.	Virtually none.
ADAPTATION	About 15 days. Wearing time critical.	About a week. Wearing time lenient.
NIGHT VISION	Often vulnerable to reflections, side glare.	Good.
PRESCRIPTION CHANGES	Reasonable amounts can be done with same lenses.	New lenses needed.
MATERIAL LIFE	Many years.	Unpredictable.
OCCUPATIONS	May pop out in contact sports. Dirt may get under lens in dirty atmosphere.	Cannot be worn where there are sprays in air, i.e., auto body shops, beauty shops, etc. Good for sports.
CHANGING FROM CONTACTS TO GLASSES	Sight not too good after removing.	No problem. Can interchange freely.
CLEANING	Simple.	Some substances may be difficult to remove.
FALLING OUT	Possible.	Very improbable.
SLIDING OFF CORNEA	Possible.	Very improbable.
DUST & DIRT	Can get under lens and irritate eye.	Almost never gets under lens.
CLIMATE	No significant difference.	May become uncomfortable in dry climates.
TINTS	Any color possible.	Only clear.
BIFOCALS & MULTIFOCALS	Available in various types.	Not available.
FITTING FEE (INCL. LENSES)	$150 to $225 (More for special lenses).	$275 to $375.

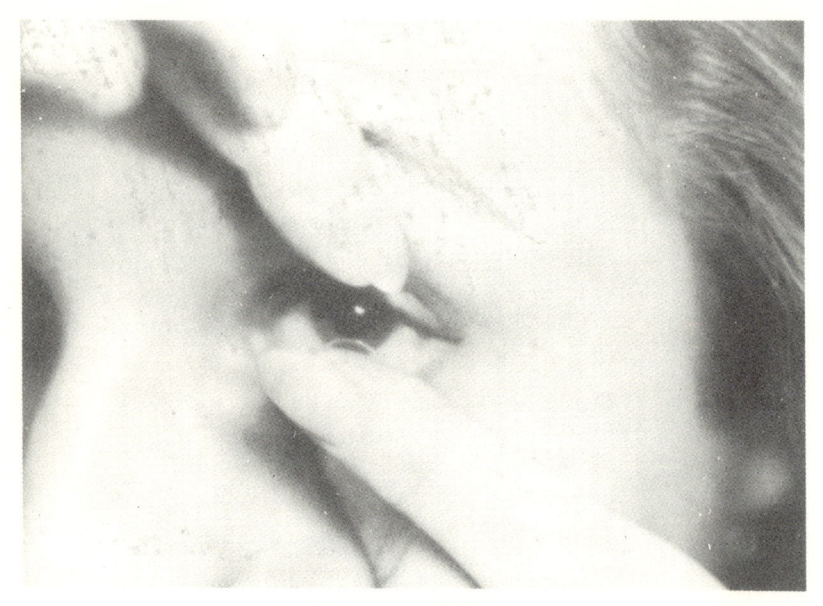

Inserting a contact lens onto the cornea.

CHAPTER 21

GUIDE TO SUCCESSFUL WEAR

We must emphasize that the indispensable ingredient for successfully wearing contact lenses is a good fitting procedure by the doctor. After that, you'll find wearing contacts is a very individual experience; you must learn to live with them. The hints and tips listed below should make it a little bit easier for you. They are not, however, intended to compensate for a poor fit.

The First Few Days

Before you leave the doctor's office with your new contacts, you should feel confident that you can put them on your eyes and take them out by yourself. You should also be able to move a displaced lens back onto the cornea. If these maneuvers give you trouble when you are at home, carefully review the instructions. You are probably doing something just a little bit wrong—turning your head, rolling your eye, etc. Just stay calm, go over the directions, and proceed slowly, step by step.

The doctor prescribed a wearing schedule which increases the daily hours of wear. Stick to it as closely as possible. Assuming you have the hard lenses, you will be aware of them much of the time. You may experience periods of considerable tearing, which will cause the lenses to move around more than they should. They may occasionally slide off the cornea onto the white part of the eye. Don't get upset. The lenses cannot go behind your eyes into your head. Simply move it back into place. If the lens will not move into place easily, and as long as it doesn't hurt, forget about it for a while. Try again later when you are calmer.

Good sunglasses are almost mandatory since you will probably be sensitive to light and glare. Frequently, there is some burning, itching, and sensation of heat. No matter how tempted you might be, DO NOT RUB YOUR EYES. As you get used to the contacts, these minor irritations gradually ease off. If they don't, report them to the doctor.

Most of the symptoms mentioned in the previous paragraph do not exist with the soft contacts. Instead, you may find your vision fluctuating from time to time. With either the hard or soft lenses, the following problems are NOT normal:

1. Inability to keep the eyes open.
2. Pain when wearing the contacts or after removing them.
3. Unbearable light sensitivity.
4. Hazy vision and/or colored rings around lights.
5. Harsh burning or severe irritation.
6. Eyes very red.

Admittedly, some of these symptoms vary only in degree from normal symptoms, but to be safe, remove the lenses and report to the doctor. Incidentally, you should have the doctor's home telephone number in case of an emergency.

Approaching Full-Time Wear

Each day you will wear the lenses a little bit longer until you reach "full-time" wear. We put that into quotes because it doesn't mean twenty-four hours a day, and it doesn't mean the same thing for all patients. Some can wear the lenses sixteen to eighteen hours a day, others less. Your doctor will guide you in this by carefully checking your eyes at regular intervals. If it turns out that your wearing time is twelve hours a day, don't despair about having to wear your glasses to a late party. Just take the contacts out for about an hour late in the afternoon, and then you can wear them another six to eight hours. (You might take a nap for that hour and be really fresh for the party.) After removing the contacts and replacing them with glasses, your sight may be blurred. This should disappear within two hours. If it takes longer, report it to the doctor.

Maintaining Schedule

Once you are wearing the contacts regularly, you should try to maintain approximately the same schedule every day. This is very important with the hard lenses, less so with the soft ones. For instance, it is unwise to wear them continually for eighteen hours if you normally only wear them for twelve. It could cause an abrasion on the cornea, which means the surface layer is scraped or scratched. You might not feel the injury while the lenses are on your eyes, but a couple of hours after taking them out, you will experience pain, intolerance to light, and copious tearing. It's one of the more unpleasant incidents in life. Call your doctor. The only consolation is that the healing process is rapid (about thirty-six hours) and complications are rare. You can take a couple of aspirins. Cold compresses over the closed lids may relieve some of the pain. Follow this by placing a tight pressure bandage over the lids to keep eye movements to a minimum. A topical anesthesia on the cornea can be used to reduce the pain, but it slows down the healing process by a few days. So, if you keep your eyes closed and suffer, the time is shortened. The doctor must check your eyes to make certain there are no complications. You will also be advised as to when you should resume wearing the contacts.

If the lenses are improperly fitted, or if you have not

worn them for a few days (perhaps due to illness or a lost lens) and then resume wearing them for a complete day, painful abrasions may also occur. To avoid any mishaps, follow this schedule:

NOT WORN	SCHEDULE
1 day	2 hours less than normal the 1st day, then normal.
2 to 3 days	8 hours the 1st day and increase 2 hours per day to normal.
3 to 5 days	6 hours the 1st day and increase 2 hours a day to normal.
More than 5 days	4 hours the 1st day and increase 1 hour a day for next 3 days, then increase 2 hours a day to normal.

With the soft contacts there is much greater leniency in the wearing schedule, and the chances of getting an abrasion are quite slim. Don't interpret this as permission to wear them excessively or erratically. Even with the soft lenses, it is best to maintain a steady, daily schedule.

Sleeping

Never wear your lenses when sleeping. A short catnap may not hurt your eyes, but short catnaps have a way of becoming longer. Supposing you do fall asleep with hard lenses. Remove them as soon as you awaken and hope you haven't injured the cornea. With the soft lenses you may wake up seeing a haze or cloudiness. This is caused by the drying of the lenses and a slight swelling of the cornea. DO NOT TRY TO REMOVE THE LENSES IMMEDIATELY; when dry, they tend to stick to the cornea. Put a few drops of saline solution into the eyes and wait a few minutes until the lenses slide freely off the cornea. You can then remove them without any complications.

Difficult Wearing Times

There are times and circumstances when the contacts may be very uncomfortable or simply not feasible. Smoky, hot rooms such as you might encounter at cocktail parties, will irritate the eyes. Other than avoiding them altogether, you might step outside every once in a while and let the eyes breathe. If the outside atmosphere is polluted, you may not get much relief. Belting down a few alcoholic drinks will tend to dry the eyes and increase the irritation.

Colds and hay fever prevent some people from being able to wear their lenses. The soft contacts are usually more tolerant under these circumstances. Some women have difficulty wearing contacts during pregnancy and have to temporarily reduce the hours or discontinue wear. Many people experience burning and haziness when reading or watching TV for a long time. Lack of eye movement and adequate blinking are the cause. Some extra blinking and occasionally looking away from the book or TV set should solve the problem.

Something In The Eye

With the hard lenses it is quite possible for a piece of soot or dirt to fall into the eye and become trapped between the lens and the cornea. A good way to get it out is to hold the upper lid firmly against the bone under the eyebrow and blink violently. If the foreign particle still remains, take the lens out, rinse it off and put it back.

With the soft lenses, once it's in place, it is nearly impossible for something to get between the cornea and the lens. But, it can happen while putting them on. Don't ignore any unusual sensation hoping it will go away. Take the lens out and rinse it as often as necessary until it feels right. A tiny hair or fragment of thread may defy several rinsings before it finally comes off. There is also the possibility that the lens may be inside-out.

Dropped Lenses

As careful as you might be, you will have your share of dropped lenses. If you insert and remove your lenses over a sink, we assume you have either stoppered the drain or placed a towel across it. Many people forget this simple precaution and find themselves playing plumber. (Once in a while the lens is found.)

If dropped, the hard lens should only be picked up by wetting a finger, touching it to the lens and lifting it straight up. Don't drag it along or you'll scratch it. Sometimes the lens lands dome side up and sticks to the surface with suction. Pour a little water over it, float it loose and slide a piece of paper under it. Never use a sharp implement to pry it loose.

The soft lens is more difficult to find because it makes no sound when it drops, is colorless, and will cling to the sides of walls and furniture. The longer it takes to find it, the more time the lens has to dry and shrivel. The lens is very brittle in this form. Pick it up with a piece of paper and rewet it before touching it. It is best not to wear a lens that you think may have been damaged until you have it checked.

Swimming, Showering, Washing And Crying

Whether you are swimming, showering, washing or crying, the common denominator is the chance of too much liquid in the eyes. It is safer not to wear contacts while swimming, unless you keep your head out of water and narrow your lids. Opening the eyes under water is a no-no. It will cause the lenses to float out of your eyes; you will have little chance of ever finding them. The soft lenses are less likely to come off, but when swimming in chlorinated water, the lenses may soak up the chlorine and irritate the eyes.

For showering or washing, you can simply shut your eyes when the water splashes on your face. Be extra careful not to get any soap in your eyes.

Some crying shouldn't affect the contacts, but if you're watching a real tear-jerker, the hard lenses may slide off the cornea.

Occasional Eyeglass Wear

There are times when you will want to wear your glasses—early in the morning, late at night, if you lose a lens, etc. You should have a pair of eyeglasses with your current prescription available.

With soft contacts, other than the normal distortions from eyeglasses, it is very easy to interchange contacts and spectacles without any visual disturbances.

Hard contacts pose a problem. After removing hard lenses, most people have difficulty seeing with glasses. This may last an hour or so. Also, your vision with glasses will vary depending on the time of day you wear them, and how long the contacts were in your eyes.

Makeup

It's almost axiomatic that a woman who has been wearing glasses and switches to contacts, begins to use more makeup. If done with care and moderation, that's perfectly all right.

Put the lenses on your eyes *before* applying the makeup. It's best to use water soluble products, and avoid getting any of them on your lenses. A particularly bothersome item is a lash lengthener which contains tiny hairlike particles. We recall seeing one soft lens that was actually pierced by one of these particles. Any makeup which gets on the lens will not only irritate the eyes, but contaminate the lenses. Because it is difficult to clean foreign matter from them, the soft contacts are very vulnerable.

Sprays of any type are not only bad for the environment in general, but terrible on contacts. If you absolutely must use a spray product, close your eyes and keep them shut for at least half a minute after spraying. In beauty shops, there is so much mist and spray in the air that it's best not to wear the lenses.

Make sure there is no makeup on your fingers when you handle the lenses. This rule also applies to certain soaps which contain lotions, creams or perfumes. Use a mild soap such as Ivory or Nutrigena.

Prescription Changes

With contact lenses there are usually fewer yearly changes in the power of the prescription than with glasses. Occasionally, changes are necessary. If the change is moderate, your hard lenses can be reground to the new power. Soft lenses cannot be reground; new contacts with the correct power must be obtained.

Scratches

Hard lenses can be scratched with careless handling. When enough scratches accumulate on the lens, its surface will not wet properly. The dry spots will cause hazy vision and some discomfort. As long as the scratches are not too deep, they can be removed by polishing.

Contact Lens Solutions

There are probably as many wetting, soaking, and cleaning solutions for hard contact lenses as there are headache remedies. Just like headache remedies, they are all supposed to do the same thing, but you may find that a particular brand works best for you. Stick with that brand, but follow the directions printed on the bottle.

Solutions for hard lenses should *never* be used with the soft lenses. You can easily ruin the lenses and irritate your eyes.

Besides wetting and cleaning solutions, there are a host of products to make your eyes more comfortable while wearing contacts. If the lenses are fitted correctly, these products are rarely needed. Most of them can only be safely used with hard lenses. Check with your doctor before using any commercial product.

Glare

With hard contacts, even after the initial adaptation period, you will tend to be a little more sensitive to bright light and glare. Use good sunglasses (see Chapter 17) whenever you are outdoors in sunshine. At night you may get some sparkle and a shimmering effect from the edge of the lenses. If it's very bothersome, the lenses may have to be adjusted or even changed. The soft lenses cause very little problem with glare, light sensitivity, or sparkle.

Continuing Care

The most important thing you can do to assure yourself of safe and comfortable wear year after year, is to have your eyes and contacts examined preferably every six months. Your eyes *do* change, whether you realize it or not. Although you may not feel it, the contacts may be causing injury to the cornea. After wearing contacts for a long time, the cornea becomes less sensitive to pain, and a serious condition may be developing without you being aware of it. Regular checkups by your doctor can head off any potential problems.

Part V

CHILDREN'S VISION

CHAPTER 22

THE DEVELOPING VISUAL SYSTEM—HOW IT MATURES

The full story on how the visual system develops is clouded and incomplete. You obviously can't ask the newborn baby what and how it sees and expect a cogent answer. Experiments are difficult to devise and carry out. Nevertheless, during the last few years great strides have been made in furthering our understanding. For instance, even though an infant uses only one eye at a time, it has been shown that its visual system is quite complete, including capabilities for full 3-dimensional vision.

One particular experiment had a very surprising result. A baby watching a moving object disappear behind a screen, fully expects it to reappear on the other side. Logically, this would seem to be a learned process, yet it is apparently built into the system. This puts a new slant on the "Peek-a-Boo" game. The baby *expects* your face to be behind your hands. He doesn't think it has disappeared. The squeal of delight is because he sees your face again, not because he is startled. However, if you keep your face hidden a long time, he will forget about it (babies have a very short memory span), and then be startled.

Other experiments have shown that the infant correlates objects with places. In other words, an apple in one location becomes a different apple when placed in another spot. He also thinks an object in motion is not the same object when it stands still. By a few months of age, however, the baby no longer has these misconceptions. As he gains more information from his own movements, the visual system probably makes the changeover.

The two parts to the big controversy are: What is built into the system, and what has to be learned. Both play an important role. Let's trace a few of the basic steps.

The space world of the infant is quite close, probably within a few feet. Most of the seeing is done with one eye at a time. When the baby is a month old, you will notice that he's able to direct both eyes at the same near object. At first these eye movements are jerky and uneven, but within a short time, they become smooth and easy. At this stage he will turn his head not only to follow moving objects, but also when changing fixation. In time he will learn to gain the same visual information by only moving his eyes.

By the age of three months, his eyes should be working as a team for seeing at all distances. Certainly by one year, the teamwork should be well developed and neither eye should go wandering off by itself. When your child is tired, should you notice that one eye seems to be turned, or worse yet, if it is constantly turned, your child needs help. If your doctor says: "Let's wait and see," find yourself another doctor. If you wait, the child *won't* see.

It's fairly easy for you to check whether the baby's eyes are working together. Hold a lighted candle about three feet away and watch the flame reflected on the cornea. The image should be centered in the black pupil at about the same position on each eye. A crossed eye cannot be ignored, nor can treatment be delayed. Failure of the two eyes to work together at an early age, will result in abnormal development and possibly amblyopia (see Chapter 24).

Most of the physical growth of the eyes occurs within the first three years of life. There seems to be an ongoing kind of compensation among the cornea, lens, and length of the eyeball. Proper development of this optical system will theoretically result in a perfectly focused image on the retina. More often than not, it doesn't work out quite that well.

If you are over forty, and have to hold your reading at

arm's length, you can envy your fourteen-year old who can see the same print at three inches from his or her eyes. At that age he or she has reached the maximum flexibility of the focusing mechanism. After that, it's downhill. The importance of this flexibility will become apparent in the Chapter 26, Reading Problems Equal School Failures.

The visual system will mature as long as light, forms, and shapes are permitted to stimulate the retina. However, all the other senses must add their input for the brain to receive the meaning. For example, is that round three-dimensional object coming at you, hard or soft, a basketball or a balloon? Touch and feel are ways the brain learns the first time around. It doesn't matter if you feel the basketball with your hands or if it bounces off your head—the brain records the information. Later, the brain can make a reasonable guess from simple visual clues. If the object floats around, the brain makes its "best bet" and chooses "balloon." Whether an object is hot or cold is a similar experience. Touch must originally be integrated into the total perception. (Many people are burned with electric irons because there are no visual clues as to whether they are hot or cold, on or off.)

There is evidence that size scaling must also be programmed into the brain with touch. Hence, when the baby "gets into" everything, hold back the scolding. He's merely working out a computer program for his brain. In addition, he is improving his hand/eye coordination.

As you may now realize, the infant can "see," but what he sees lacks meaning. He slowly builds a meaningful world by integrating all the other senses. Not to be overlooked when we speak of senses, is the movement of his body and the resulting feedback. This supplies the brain with much information, i.e., how far he is from an object, and where the object is in relation to another. Only by physically moving from one place to another can he learn to later judge distances with visual clues only. Put these things all together and they spell vision, or more aptly, perception.

CHAPTER 23

THE EXAMINATION OF THE INFANT AND PRE-SCHOOLER

For reasons which will become obvious to you in the next few chapters, the vision and eye health problems of the infant and pre-schooler must be detected early. We strongly urge that every child be seen routinely by an optometrist beginning at the age of two years, and much earlier if there is a family history of vision or eye problems.

These examinations are most important because the child cannot tell you if something is wrong. As far as the child is concerned, it's the normal way to see. Most parents rely heavily on the advice of the pediatrician to make certain that the child's visual development is normal. However, with the exception of the obvious problems which you may even notice yourself, the pediatrician is not really knowledgeable in vision and eye care. This is not meant to condemn the pediatrician. This particular doctor is so busy coping with fevers, innoculations, injuries, allergies, runny noses, and aching tummies that even if he or she knew the special procedures, there is probably little time for a full vision evaluation. Therefore, parents dare not assume a child is seeing correctly without a proper optometric examination.

What do we look for when we examine this young child? First, we observe the child's general posture, how he or she moves, if he or she favors one side of the body. Then, concentrating on the eyes, we check the response of the pupils to light, inspect the outside of the eyes, the lids, and the inside of the eyes for any signs of possible disease or abnormality.

When we have established that the eyes are healthy, we begin a series of vision tests. We give top priority to the two eyes working together when the child looks at different distances. We observe if the eyes are able to converge—turn inward—when an object is held close, and if the eyes diverge smoothly when the object is removed and the child must look far away. Neither eye should show any tendency to cross.

Frequently, parents bring a child into the office because they have a complaint that goes something like this: "Doctor, I think Susie has a crossed eye." If the examination confirms that it actually is a crossed eye, special tests will determine if it is crossed occasionally, constantly, the degree and direction of crossing, etc. This information helps in deciding the type of therapy that will be prescribed. If, on the other hand, the examination results show the eyes to be straight, most likely the parents' observations were faulty. This is understandable if the child's nose bridge structure is flat and not yet fully developed. If this is the case, even normal eye movements can give the false appearance of a crossed eye. We cannot overlook the possibility, however, that the child's eyes may cross only when he or she is tired. We advise the parents to observe the child carefully and return for a retesting.

Another part of the examination is a subjective check of the visual acuity. It is possible to do this with a very young child, even though the child cannot read any letters. Admittedly, it's a challenge and requires some patience. We use the tiny sugar pellets sprinkled on cakes for decorations. The size of these pellets is about 1/25th of an inch, and we place them on a white cloth, twelve or fourteen inches in front of the child. Covering one eye at a time, we watch how quickly the child can spot and pick them up. It is not accurate, but certainly indicates if the child has

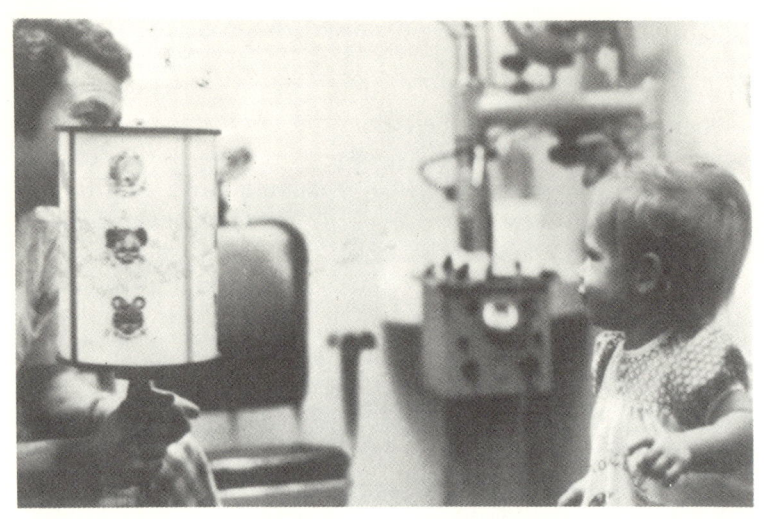

The rotating optokinetic drum can determine the child's visual acuity objectively.

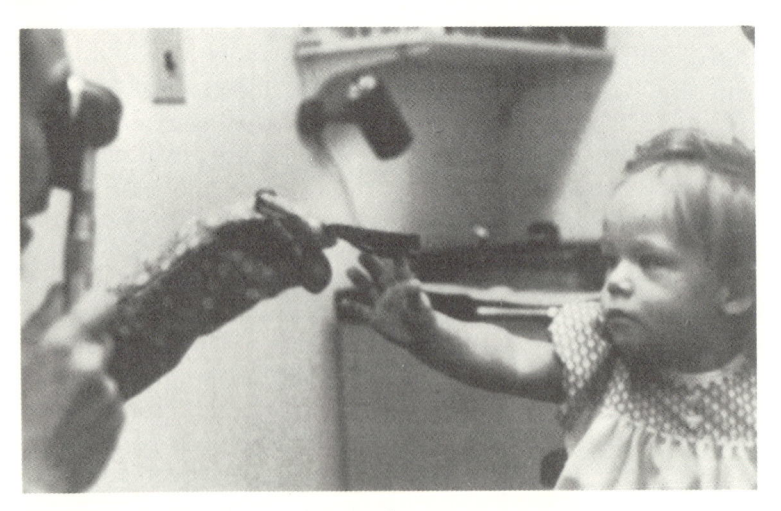

The hand puppet keeps the child's attention while using the retinoscope.

reasonably good sight in each eye, and particularly if he or she sees about the same with each eye. Of course, the child is allowed to eat any sugar pellets he or she picks up—a privilege not granted to the examining doctor or the parents. You can try this simple test with your child at home.

As the child gets older, we may use familiar objects such as toys and animal pictures to determine the visual acuity. When he or she is old enough to know directionality, we will use the tumbling E. This is the letter E facing in different directions.

Passing the simple subjective acuity test is no guarantee that the child does not have astigmatism, nor does it totally rule out farsightedness or nearsightedness. Actually, we can, and do detect these problems completely objectively, without any direct responses from the child. This surprises some parents, but it's really rather easy for the experienced optometrist. By using an instrument called a retinoscope to look into the eyes, we can readily determine any refractive condition. The same instrument is used to measure the focusing ability of the eyes. We are particularly watchful that the eyes are focusing equally and directly on the target.

Before the child enters kindergarten, we will include tests for depth perception and color vision. We want to catch the child with a color vision deficiency so that we may alert the school. Teachers are very fond of using color-coded material as teaching aids. Imagine the difficulties the child with an undetected color vision problem will have.

If we find everything to be normal, everyone is happy. But, remember that your child is growing, the eyes are changing and visual requirements become more demanding. A yearly examination is, therefore, highly advisable.

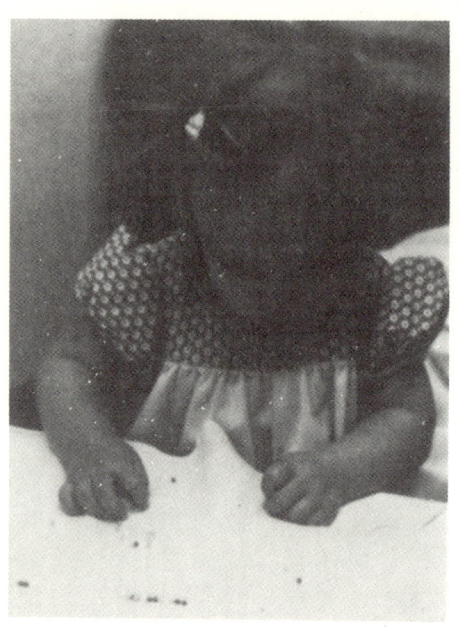

Small sugar pellets can be used to test the child's seeing ability.

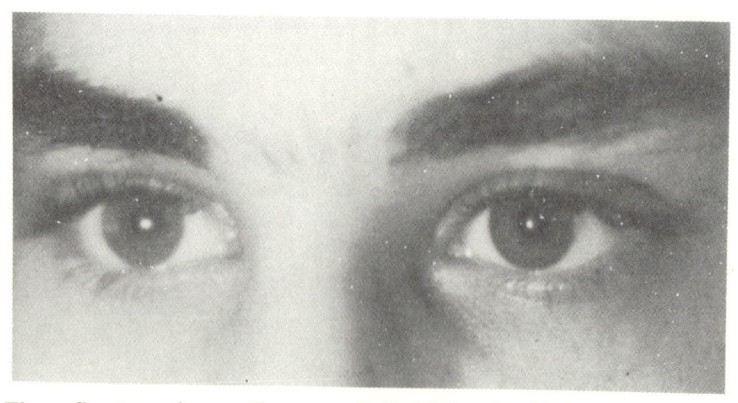

The reflection of a candle or small flashlight should be centered in the pupil of each eye.

SYMPTOMS WHICH MAY INDICATE VISUAL PROBLEMS IN YOUR CHILD

1. Rubbing the eyes.
2. Headaches, especially after reading.
3. Closing or covering one eye.
4. Squinting when looking at the chalkboard.
5. Avoidance of close work, reading.
6. Tilting the head to one side.
7. Holding reading material very close.
8. Losing place while reading.
9. Moving the head instead of eyes when reading.
10. Persistent letter or word reversal after the second grade.
11. Confusing similar words.
12. Frequently leaving out words.
13. Hyperactivity.
14. Persistent motion (car) sickness.
15. Awkwardness.
16. Blurring of vision at any time.

The visual causes for many of these symptoms are not readily picked up in a typical school screening test. The value of the screening is limited, and it should *never* be construed to be a vision examination.

CHAPTER 24

AMBLYOPIA—"LAZY EYE"

What is a "lazy" eye? Can you have two "lazy" eyes? Have you ever heard of a "lazy" ear or a "lazy" finger? What is so unique about the visual system that permits the condition of amblyopia or "lazy" eye?

The word "amblyopia" comes from the Greek, meaning dull vision. In modern usage it generally refers to a particular type of dull vision; there is no detectable disease, and sight is not fully correctable with lenses.

There are basically two types of amblyopia: The first is caused by toxic substances such as alcohol or tobacco, and the second is caused by lack of use.

A careful case history of the patient is often the best clue as to which type we are dealing with. The one we are concerned with here is amblyopia "ex-anopsia" (a fancy term for lack of use). This type makes up the majority of cases, is found frequently in children, and presents the greatest challenge for treatment.

On the face of it, not using an eye seems ridiculous. The eye is open so it must be seeing. However, as the old song goes, "It Ain't Necessarily So." With both eyes open, which eye are you seeing with? Do you see equally well with both eyes? (You might be surprised at the number of people who have never compared the sight of their two eyes. Patients who are being examined for the first time are frequently amazed when we show them the difference in what each eye sees.)

Minute differences anywhere along the path of light rays in the eye can be very significant. For instance, an increase of the length of the eyeball of *only 1 mm* (about 1/25th of an inch) can plunge visual acuity from 20/20 to 20/400. To provide the best sight with stereoscopic vision, the two eyes have to work together in exquisite balance. What do you suppose happens when something interferes with those balances?

Instead of receiving equal information from the two eyes, suppose the brain, for reasons we will discuss shortly, receives different information from each eye. There is an old adage used in computer technology called GIGO. This means—garbage in, garbage out. If you feed nonsense into a computer, nonsense answers will emerge. If you feed conflicting information into the brain, a similar situation exists.

But, the brain is cleverer than a computer. Since the sense of vision is so vital and since the brain is so dependent on it, the two different inputs will not be tolerated. Let's face it, if there is one tree in your path and each eye signals the brain that it is in a different place or distance, you are liable to run right into that tree. This is hardly healthy for the organism.

The brain will gladly sacrifice the benefits of stereoscopic vision to avoid the dreadful confusion of double vision. It simply learns to ignore the input from one eye. This is not all that difficult. If, while you are reading this, you hold the palm of your hand about three inches in front of one eye, you can continue to read even if you are vaguely aware of the hand. If you did it long enough, the awareness of your hand would become less and less. The brain is simply ignoring the visual input of the covered eye. If you did this for a very long time (a child growing up with the input being ignored for many years), the pattern would become so ingrained, that a normal binocular pattern may not be established or may even be lost. Then, even if the original cause of the problem was removed, the brain could not reestablish binocular vision by itself. It would need help, and that's where visual therapy for amblyopia comes in.

Why would the two eyes feed different information to the brain? As we mentioned before, the difference in the size of the two eyeballs could be one reason. It's not all that unusual, either, when you consider that your two feet or two ears are probably not identical in size. If the brain receives one clear and one blurry image, it will latch on to the clear one and disregard the blurred one. Other causes of unequal sight will have similar results.

Almost invariably, amblyopia goes together with eyes that are turned in or out. Which comes first? It can happen either way. Suppose the blurry image is stubborn about being ignored. The brain then has a choice of turning the eye so that the image falls on a less discriminating part of the retina, or better still, on the natural blind spot, to solve the problem. Or, it may happen another way. If the eyes are very farsighted, in order to see clearly at distance, the eyes must resort to using a tremendous amount of lens focusing. This also causes the eyes to turn inward. (Normally, the focusing is only called into play to see objects up close. Then the eyes *should* turn in to keep the target centered on the foveas.) Since these two functions are linked by nerve impulses and do not work independently, the net result is that distant objects will be seen double. This dilemma will not be tolerated by the brain; amblyopia and/or crossed eyes will result.

There are other scenarios possible with many complicating variations, but the idea is the same. Amblyopia is one of the brain's solutions to an insufferable situation. It comes down to this: The brain will go to almost any lengths to avoid double vision.

Can this condition be corrected? Frequently it can, depending on the particular cause, but it requires a lot of persistence. First of all, special tests must be taken to determine the specific problem. Is the eye looking straight at the target object? Does the amplyopic eye show a greater need for corrective lenses? Is one eye sighting higher or lower than the other? Is the nerve pathway from the macula to the brain complete? Is there a blind spot (other than the normal one)? There are many possibilities.

Treatment will depend on the results of these tests. Generally, the procedure will follow three stages:

1. Correction of the sight problem with glasses or contact lenses.
2. Some type of concentrated stimulation to the macula of the amblyopic eye.
3. Straightening the eye if it is turned, and building binocular, stereoscopic vision with the eyes working together.

It is a long process requiring diligent work by the patient. The longer the problem has existed, the more difficult the remediation. If you remember nothing else in this chapter, engrave this on your memory: Children don't "grow out" of this condition, they grow more severely into it. Early detection is the best way of avoiding additional complications.

CHAPTER 25

CROSSED EYES

The expressions "cross-eyed," "wall-eyed," "squint," "cock-eyed," "tropia," and "strabismus," all refer to the same disorder—one eye does not point in the same direction as the other. In ancient times people with crossed eyes were thought to be bewitched, and were subsequently treated with cruelty. We are a little more sophisticated now; we only make these people subjects of ridicule and the butt of jokes. Naturally, cross-eyed people are sensitive about their looks, but the look is only the visible symptom of a deeper problem.

You probably think of crossed eyes as looking at each other. Actually, they can assume many forms. One eye may turn up or down, in or out, even a combination such as in with up, etc. The eye may also be crossed constantly or only occasionally. You may be tempted to ignore the occasional crossing of your child's eye, but don't!

In all cases of strabismus, one eye does the sighting while the other eye looks somewhere else. In a few people, the sighting eye and the turning eye alternate roles, i.e., sometimes the right and sometimes the left will turn away.

A common misconception is that crossed eyes are caused by weak muscles. The muscles attached to the eye are very strong and the range of movement is quite remarkable. You can easily follow moving objects, rapidly shift your gaze, and imitate Eddie Cantor by rolling your eyes in a circle. Except in rare cases, even crossed eyes are able to move freely *one at a time.* If you cover the sighting eye, the turned eye will swing into sighting position and make all the movements. For various reasons, the two eyes just won't work *together;* they won't look at the same object at the same time.

An eye can become crossed because of some hereditary defect or birth injury, a paralyzed muscle, or disease of the nervous system. But, all of theses reasons taken together represent only a small fraction of squint cases we encounter. The majority of crossed eyes are due to some functional disorder. By that we mean that the brain doesn't order the eyes to coordinate their movements and work together.

Why would the brain refuse to coordinate the action of the two eyes? The most likely explanation seems to be the brain's desire to avoid double vision. This can happen, of course, if the separate images from the two eyes are radically different. The brain will go to any lengths to see singly, even if it means supressing the sight of one eye.

One of the most frequent types of crossed eyes that we encounter is linked to high amounts of farsightedness. This is the classic case of one eye turning inward toward the nose. The probable sequence of events runs like this: To see clearly, the farsighted eye must use an extraordinary amount of focusing power. But, since focusing and turning the eyes inward work together, the eyes will turn too much and ultimately, will cross.

Other types of crossed eyes have other causes; we do not know all the reasons. The optometrist is faced with the task of determining the type and degree. This requires rather extensive, specialized testing. A careful history of the patient is quite important; in some families there is a strong hereditary tendency toward crossed eyes. Usually, several members will exhibit it to varying degrees.

Once the condition is diagnosed, the optometrist will embark on a program to straighten the eyes. The eye which crosses occasionally is the easiest to deal with and, provided it is discovered early, treatment results are very favorable. At this early stage, parents usually ignore the condition and hope it will go away by itself. It hardly ever does, of course, and can become an amblyopic eye. If the eye does become amblyopic, we have to deal with two conditions, making therapy much more difficult.

We will not go into the actual therapy procedures, but the following are the logical steps to be taken over a period of months.

First, glasses are prescribed; sometimes even bifocals for children. If necessary, we'll incorporate a prism effect into the lenses to shift the images closer together.

When amplyopia is present, we have to break up the supression habit; then the patient is actually made aware of seeing double when the eyes are not straight. Next, the patient is trained to fuse the two images into one. As this progresses, the eyes will become straighter. Finally, depth perception is developed and the new seeing pattern strengthened to keep the eyes from recrossing.

If these methods don't work, then surgery may be indicated. But, in the vast majority of cases, surgery should be the *last* resort—not the first one. A functional cure through therapy is more natural than the procedure of violent surgical intervention. There are always risks involved when any surgery is performed. If it's the only option left, visual therapy must also be provided to help the eyes function together, as well as to prevent any future crossing.

The alternating crossed eyes are the most difficult to correct, even though amblyopia is rarely present. Generally, the alternating pattern seems to be deeply imbedded in the brain's visual system and resists visual therapy remediation. At that point, muscle surgery, followed by visual therapy is the only recourse.

If you remember nothing else from this chapter, remember this: If your child's eyes cross, visit your family optometrist promptly! Don't wait for your child to complain. There is usually no discomfort with a crossed eye (except the taunts of other children). Don't ignore it just because it seems to be only a small amount of crossing or it only happens occasionally. It may not look bad cosmetically, but visually it's just as bad as an eye turned all the way in or out. Even a small amount of squint interferes with normal three-dimensional vision and will hamper the person later in life.

CHAPTER 26

READING PROBLEMS EQUAL SCHOOL FAILURES

This subject is very controversial and quite complex. Like the common cold, there are many theories and many "cures." But, unlike the common cold which you get rid of in seven days with or without treatment, a child with a reading disability is not likely to get rid of it in a week, a year or a lifetime. The child is trapped in a world of academic defeats, frustration and school failures which translate into an antipathy to school. He often defies his teachers and parents whom he subconsciously blames for putting him into an unpleasant situation.

As you will learn later in this chapter, the act of reading is very intricate and requires meticulous coordination of many physical and mental processes, beginning in the eye and ending in the brain. When we examine poor readers, we consistently find lapses in one or more of these interrelated functions.

Common eyesight problems, when they are found, must be corrected with glasses or contact lenses. But, there are more causes for problems than nearsightedness, farsightedness or astigmatism. A typical fault is that the child has trouble in smoothly moving both eyes together in all directions. He will move his head instead of his eyes. You can watch the child yourself and ascertain if this is happening, but you cannot tell if there is a flaw in the focusing mechanism which is supposed to keep the print clear. Nor can you tell if both eyes are looking (converging) at the same place on the page.

Any shortcomings in these aptitudes will cause fatigue when reading. The normal response to fatigue or stress is to stop the activity that is causing it; ergo, the child won't read for more than a few minutes.

Not all children respond in the same way to fatigue or stress. Some will push themselves and continue reading. One option they have is for the brain to shut off the sight from one eye. If they succeed completely, they may gain comfort (at the expense, perhaps, of a crossed or amblyopic eye). Usually, though, the eye will only stay shut off for a fraction of a second, or a few seconds at the most. This, of course, causes even more fatigue and a continuous vicious circle.

Sometimes the desire to use one eye is less subtle: The child reads while a hand covers one eye or the head is turned to block off vision on one side.

At the roots of these predicaments are binocular vision problems—the two eyes are simply not working as a team. Unfortunately, such a defect doesn't have a sign on it saying: "Hey, I'm faulty!" It must be searched out and tested. This is the first hurdle you as parents must cross. You would think that having the child's eyes examined would uncover binocular problems. However, this is not the case. Discovering the defect is dependent upon the proper examination.

If you take your child to an ophthalmologist who routinely uses "drops," the chances for discovering this defect are, indeed, very slim. The "drops" paralyze the eye's focusing ability—one of the functions which must be tested. You may as well audition a pianist by putting handcuffs on him! Compounding this error in examination, the other important binocular functions are usually left untested.

If you have gone this route and the ophthalmologist told you that the child *sees* fine, you have reason to be suspicious. It's like telling you that your health is fine without checking your blood pressure. Does high blood pressure not exist if the doctor fails to test for it?

On the other hand, an optometrist's examination will test to find out how the two eyes normally work together in the child's everyday world. For a proper diagnosis, the examination must include tests for eye movements, eye focusing, eye convergence, the ability to change direction of gaze easily, and whether both eyes are working together at all times, i.e., without suppression.

At present, there are many definitions for reading problems being tossed around. The terms "dyslexia" and "minimal brain dysfunction" have become fashionable descriptions for reading and learning disabilities. Rather than get bogged down in tight definitions, we will describe a typical child with this problem. Please understand that we are confining ourselves to the largest category of reading failures—that of the normally intelligent child who is behind in his expected reading level.

The pronoun "he" is quite apt here since the chances are much greater that the reading-problemed child will be a boy. (Statistically, it's at least five to one.) The reason is not hard to understand. The visual system has to reach a certain level of maturation to be ready for reading. Girls mature at an earlier age which gives them an edge. A boy who has any tendency for a reading problem will be further hampered by his slower development.

Our sample boy has an attention span that is very limited in the classroom. He is so active that he never seems to sit still. He does not get along well with his teachers or his classmates, possibly because of his hyperactivity. To quiet the child down, some pediatricians will prescribe drugs, an absolutely abhorrent practice. At the other extreme is the child who sits passively in his own world and turns off much of the classroom activity. This child has one advantage: Since he doesn't bother anyone, he is not drugged into a stupor.

In the early grades, this boy has a hard time drawing simple geometric forms. His reading is quite bad, and suffers from some of the following problems: Not reading from left to right; not being able to keep his place; leaving out words or letters; reversing words such as "was" and "saw"; confusing letters that differ only in direction, such as *p* and

q; blurred vision at near; headaches; double vision.

His general schoolwork will be poor or failing, putting a "dummy" label on him. But, take him out of the school situation or engage him in a conversation, and he will seem quite bright. His parents are convinced that he is smart (rightfully so), and blame the teachers for his reading and school failures.

After he has gone through several teachers without any reading improvement, the parents are quite puzzled. They may even decide to teach the child to read at home or to engage a tutor. Sometimes it helps, but often these tutoring sessions wind up as shouting matches with both sides frustrated. The child hardly needs another defeat.

He will try to preserve some feeling of self-worth by subconsciously covering up his failures—he will voice dislikes for school and reading. ("Who needs it? It's dumb!") As the child becomes sulky and unmanageable, the parents will begin a doctor-to-doctor merry-go-around to find out if there is some physical basis for the problems. The general physician will pass the buck to the neurologist, pediatrician, or ophthalmologist. Or, the chain may start at another point. In any event, they will all report that the child has no physical problem, may label him as having a perceptual handicap, collect their fees, and say goodbye. This leaves the parents precisely where they started.

Estimates of the number of children with these symptoms vary from 10% to 20%. That's an awful lot of kids. Thankfully, not every child shows every symptom, but even a few are enough to drive parents to distraction. The big question is—what can be done?

No matter what else you do, make sure that the child's binocular eye functions are carefully evaluated during an optometric examination. There are sound reasons why we seem to be harping on binocular eye functions. Uncovering and correcting them are probably the key to reversing the child's downward spiral. Let's take a closer look at reading and try to figure out what can go wrong.

Of course, you realize that reading is a highly artificial task imposed by our civilization. There is nothing "natural" about it, any more than there is anything "natural" in playing the piano. Evolution is not concerned with the ability to depress keys in a certain sequence. Neither is evolution concerned with the ability to recognize squiggles and lines as letters and words. The difference is that few of us must play the piano—all of us need to read.

It is generally agreed that reading is composed of three stages—reception, recognition, and comprehension. It all begins in the eye, with an image received on the retinas. These images must be clear, undistorted, and should match closely in size and shape (see Aniseikonia). Glasses or contact lenses may have to be worn for this to be accomplished.

Since reading is done within arm's reach, the eyes must focus to that distance. If the page is fourteen inches away, the focus should not be vague at thirteen or fifteen inches. To use the movie projector simile from an earlier chapter, you know that every time you move the screen closer or further, the focus must be adjusted. In the same fashion, the brain must constantly direct focusing adjustments to the eyes to keep the reading material sharp and clear.

Normally, children have a very flexible focusing system and need to use only a fraction of the total available flexibility. We consider the unused portion as being held in "reserve." However, when using both eyes together, a few children seem to be burdened with having to use all of their "reserve" to see the print. The difference here can be likened to a stroll versus running. Such a child will fatigue after a very short reading time.

Let's suppose that the focusing is good. That's just not enough. The eyes must point precisely at the words in a smooth left to right sequence (right to left for Hebrew), with a minimum of head turning. Moreover, both eyes must look at the same spot at the same time. You may think this is automatic, but many times it is not. It involves close tolerances between signals from the brain and the muscles

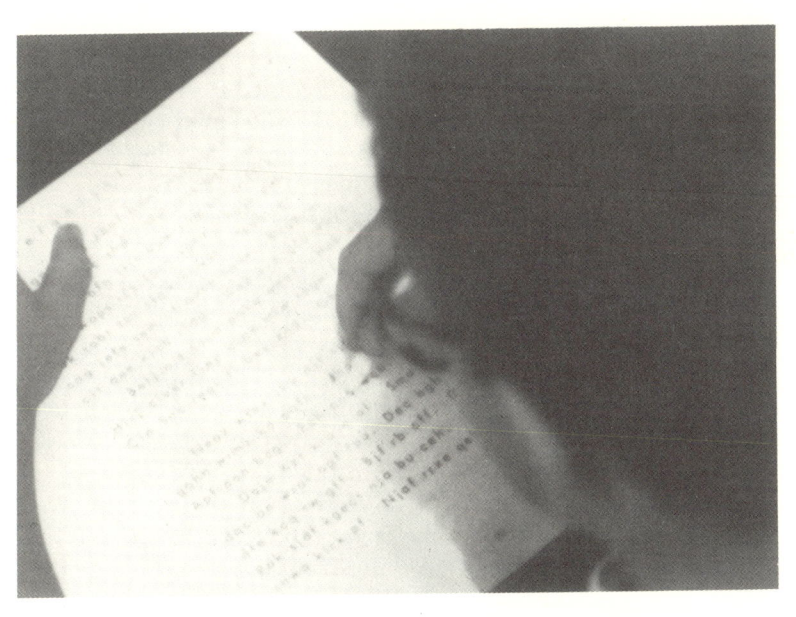

Some of the procedures used in vision therapy.

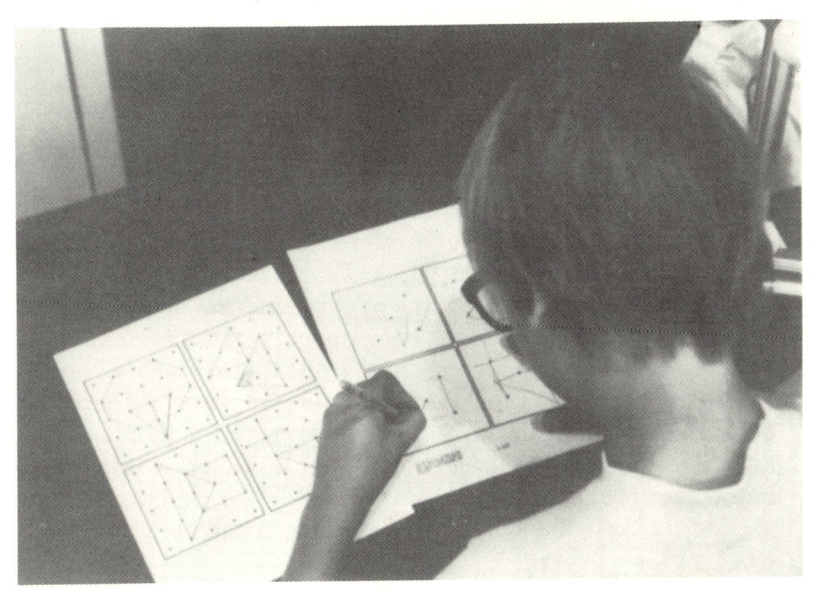

which actually move the eyes. A very slight problem with the signals from the brain or with any of the twelve muscles involved, can cause one eye to point a bit off target. Besides sweeping back and forth to read, the eyes must also converge—turn inward—to look at the print. It takes a lot of energy to sustain this convergence. As with focusing, if convergence has to be sustained for a given time at full capacity, fatigue will set in.

The second stage in reading is recognition of the nerve signals from the retina as letters and words. How does this work? Experimental evidence shows that the process in the brain for recognizing written language is very different from recognizing pictures. A picture on the retina, either a live scene or a photograph, is stored directly in the brain's memory. Written words must go through a couple of steps.

The step we're mainly concerned with here is the one-quarter of a second that it takes certain brain cells to "recognize" the word. If anything from inside or outside the body intrudes during the critical one-quarter second, the word is not "recognized." In this case, you would be aware of seeing something, but you wouldn't be able to identify it.

What do we mean by something intruding? Think of it as interference, such as static or extraneous material. For example, suppose you're reading and your mind wanders to other thoughts. Before you realize it, you're at the bottom of the page without remembering a word of what you read. That's internal interference. If you substitute a radio or a conversation, that's outside interference.

These occurrences have happened to everyone, but what we're really concerned with here is internal interference caused by visual problems. For instance, a fatigued focusing system may cause a blur during the one-quarter second, and the word is missed. The same thing can happen if the two eyes are not pointing at the same spot and a momentary different image is sent to the brain. In other words, any binocular problem can easily intrude itself as "noise."

For the sake of simplicity, we've been talking about one

word being recognized during the one-quarter second. Actually, a fast reader will recognize several words or an entire phrase, while a slow reader may only recognize a part of one word. (Speed reading courses simply teach you to recognize more words with each glance.)

Based on our clinical experience, we believe many poor readers have visual problems interfering with the recognition phase. Remember, we said *visual* problems, not *sight* problems. A *sight* problem exists only when an unclear image is formed on the retina (blurry or distorted). It is the initial reception stage of reading. A *visual* problem spans eye movements, balance, focusing, reserve energy, supressions, binocularity, and all the things which could interfere with the recognition of the printed word.

Once you get past the recognition stage, the final stage in reading is comprehension. Here the meaning and past experience of the word come together for interpretation of ideas. Thus, "ice cream" is not simply the letters i,c,e, c,r,e,a,m, but dessert, a particular flavor, a temperature, and so on. The word "tiropita" is probably Greek to you.

The prodigious comprehension stage is another realm which could be causing the child's difficulties. An increasing number of optometrists are extending their professional services to cover this field under the name of "developmental vision," or "developmental optometry." Some practitioners simply use the general term "children's vision." Whatever the nomenclature, they encompass the areas of visual performance, learning disabilities, perceptual problems, and vision training. Disparate as they may seem, there is a common bond—the concept that total vision develops through a learning process.

As was pointed out earlier, all the basic functions are built in. However, to fully develop, enrich, and give meaning to vision, experience is indispensable. During the early years of the child's growth, the brain integrates vision with the other senses and gradually *substitutes* vision for the other senses. For example, you can look at a pineapple and your brain can

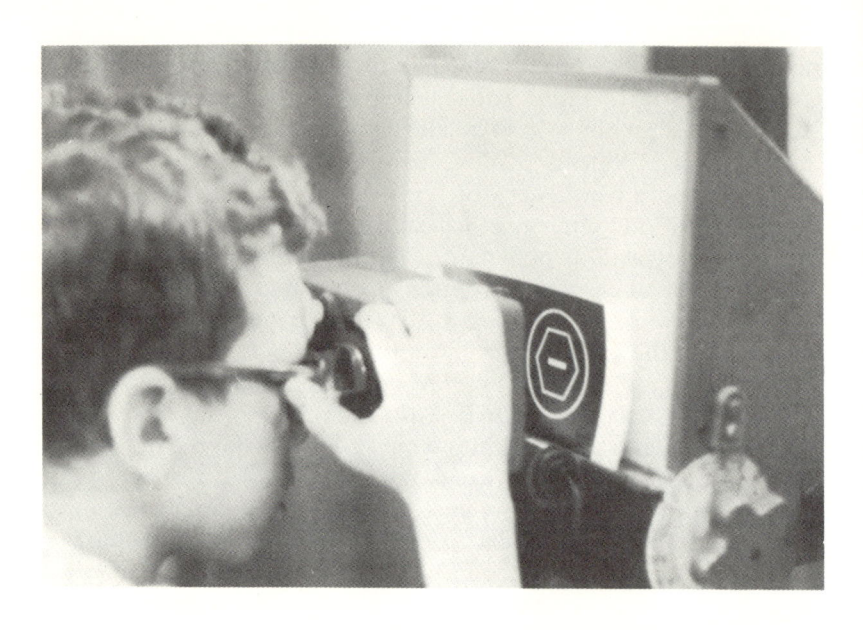

Some of the instruments used in vision therapy.

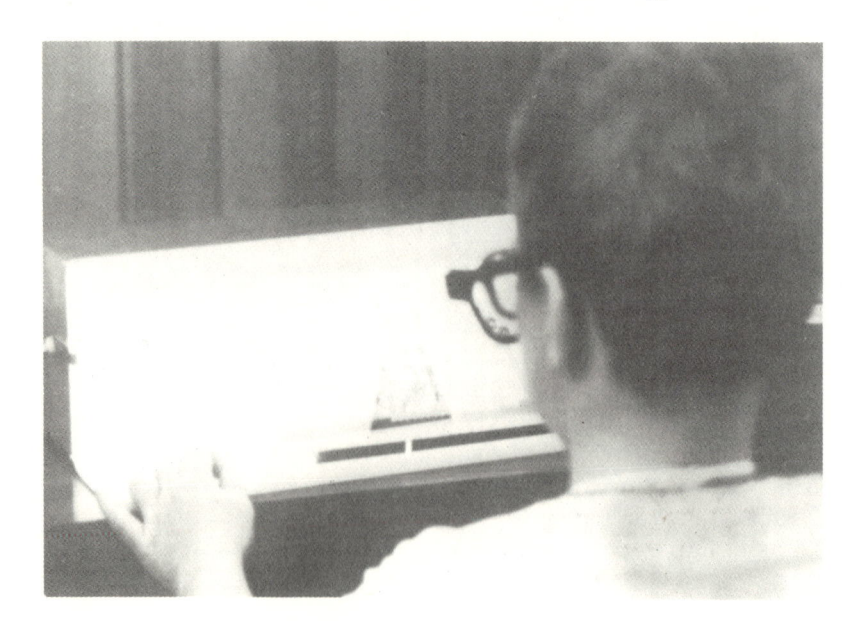

"feel" the texture and "taste" the flavor, *provided* you have previously touched and tasted it. This mental manipulation is developed through experience, and is fully interchangeable with the other senses. Hearing the word, reading the word, or thinking the word should also trigger a visual image—a sound, a touch, a taste.

Such mental maneuvering is programmed into the brain through coordination of the various senses. What are some of the things the infant or young child must learn to coordinate? Gross motor movement is probably one of the earliest, harmonizing arm, leg, and body motions—turning, sitting up, crawling, etc. With increased control of the large muscles, fine motor movements come into play for more precise hand and finger manipulation (and beginning speech). At the same time, vision is soaking up information from the surrounding space and correlating it with movement so that the child learns directionality and space concepts.

If he wants to get at a piece of candy, his vision will tell him: "Psst, it's to the left," and direct his gross and fine motor movements to the target. It he's developed good hand/eye coordination, the candy will be snatched up easily. Obviously, vision is the main steering mechanism for movement. It does yet another remarkable thing—it *replaces* movement by telling him: "Don't bother going, it's not a piece of candy." Can you appreciate the great economy of energy in learning to obtain information visually instead of having to touch the object every time? (There are times, however, when the visual information is inadequate. For example, touching a cloth surface to determine its texture.)

Learning to read complicates matters for the brain because objects and scenes are replaced with a code. The inter-sense rapport must still take place except, as pointed out earlier, additional deciphering steps are needed. In dealing with letters and words, it is particularly important to have a good visual concept of forms, shapes, and direction.

When we are faced with a child who is a poor reader, has a learning disability, or whatever you prefer to call it, we are often dealing with a child whose normal development is incomplete or muddled. Perhaps the concept of directionality is not firmly established, so that the difference between the letters "b" and "d" is not obvious. Perhaps he didn't learn to fully integrate touch with vision. Instead of gaining information about his surroundings from his vision, he has to touch objects, wasting time and energy. (This is dramatically highlighted with a severely retarded child. When presented with an unfamiliar object, he will promptly put it into his mouth, taste being a very primitive sense.) If a child cannot obtain information by looking directly at an object, how can he obtain information from a symbolized code representing that object?

We can further conjecture that the problem originated with his auditory integration, fine motor control of eye movements, spatial relationships, or any of the other systems with which the brain has dealings. Frequently, there was a lost development stage or stages in the early years of the child's life. This, of course, is a powerful reason for a professional visual analysis at an early age. Even though the brain is like a very sophisticated computer, if the programming or feed-in is faulty, it will put out unreliable answers.

Fortunately, input and programming can be corrected. Since visual functions and integration functions are learned and developed, proper relearning is possible through therapy.

Educators and psychologists are well aware of these learned processes. Many schools have incorporated gross and fine motor training into physical education programs. That's fine as far as it goes, but it's not the complete answer. Psychologists know how to test a child and categorize the developmental stage to a fine degree, but then what? Few psychologists will undertake anything but emotional problem cases. If it's a visual and/or visual perceptual problem, it will be referred to an eye practitioner. But, if the child is sent to one not versed in developmental vision, the referral is useless.

The developmental vision optometrist will both test and

train the child. This does not mean he or she will teach the child to read—that remains in the province of the educator. The optometrist will set the stage, however, by altering poor sensory patterns into smooth, coordinated signals which will pass the information to the brain where it can be properly "computed."

The relearning process is done with lenses and/or prisms, and/or training, to restructure visual, oculomotor, gross motor, and fine motor systems. Once the child is freed from the burdens of interferences created by muddled sense integrations and wasted energy, the capacity for learning to read, as well as all other forms of learning, is wide open. The rest is up to the child and the teacher. Most kids will take full advantage of their new-found skills and show remarkable improvements.

One of the joys of working with these youngsters is watching the transformation. The boy who had to touch everything in the office on his first visit, does it less and less as the training progresses. Parents are quick to notice that the child is calmer and will sustain interest in a task, instead of fitfully jumping from one thing to another.

It might be worth while to repeat that in this chapter we are talking about the "normal" child. We won't get into a debate on what "normal" means, but obviously if the child has severe emotional or mental problems, psychological help must be sought; if a hearing problem exists, auditory evaluation must be pursued. Some unfortunate children are saddled with several overlapping disorders. These are factors outside the realm of vision.

There is a valuable movement towards more interdisciplinary cooperation among all the professionals involved. This is an excellent trend, and we heartily applaud the exchange of information. Sometimes the optometrist will request an evaluation from other professionals to aid in the diagnosis.

The cooperative concept may be carried to an unnecessary extreme in "multi-disciplinary learning clinics" which house all the specialists—pediatrician, optometrist, psychologist, reading specialist, neurologist, audiologist, therapist, nutritionist, etc.—under one roof. The child makes the rounds and everyone gets into the act. When more is known about the brain's learning process and we can pinpoint the exact dysfunction, this multi-disciplinary approach will surely be discarded. At the present time, however, we feel that too much help is certainly better than no help at all. Let your optometrist be your guide.

You will discover that it is difficult to find an optometrist who is skillful in the field of learning. Hopefully, the information in this chapter will let you know when you have found the right practitioner.

CHAPTER 27

BIFOCALS FOR CHILDREN

You know that grandma and grandpa wear bifocals, and if you have reached the age when reading is difficult, you may also be wearing them. But, have you ever heard of kids wearing bifocals?

Bifocals are usually associated with older people whose ability to focus their vision on near objects such as are encountered in reading and sewing, gradually decreases. The reason, as you may recall from an earlier chapter, is that over the years, the lens of the eye slowly loses its elasticity. You may also recall from an earlier chapter that children between the ages of ten and fifteen have very flexible focusing ability. Why then would it ever be necessary to prescribe bifocals for kids?

There are four possible reasons:
1. When the ability to focus with both eyes is poor.
2. To prevent the possible crossing of one eye.
3. As a possible therapeutic measure to slow down the rapid increase of nearsightedness.
4. When the focusing is weakened because of disease or medication, or entirely missing.

First, let's consider the child who, because of poor focusing ability with the two eyes together, has difficulty reading. This child may complain that print blurs or doubles; he may have headaches or eyestrain after reading longer than a few minutes. Or, his parents might bring him into the office because he is doing poorly in school and dislikes reading.

The examining optometrist will find some test results which are fairly typical in these cases. When each eye is tested separately, the focusing ability will be normal, but when the eyes work together, the focusing is much reduced! To solve this dilemma, the child needs reading glasses for his close work. However, these reading glasses will make distant vision quite blurry, and he must take them off to see the chalkboard. It becomes an awful nuisance to constantly put the glasses on and take them off; the child will wind up not wearing them at all. A happy solution is the bifocal which allows him to see distant objects clearly through the upper half, and the reading clearly through the lower.

As well as this works, we do not consider it a permanent solution. The use of the bifocals should be accompanied by visual therapy to improve the natural focusing. Once this has been accomplished, the bifocals should no longer be needed.

Another need for bifocals will occur in the case of one eye being crossed in towards the nose, either constantly or occasionally. The bifocals make it possible to keep the eyes straight and functioning together. We might also prescribe bifocals when the examination reveals that one eye can potentially cross. Again, this is a therapeutic measure to be used while therapy is being carried on.

Let us now consider the nearsighted child who needs frequent changes to ever stronger glasses. This child is usually an excellent reader and enjoys school. But, as the nearsightedness progresses, the glasses are continually getting thicker. There is one body of opinion which feels that the increase in nearsightedness is caused by a cramping of the focusing muscles when reading. It is reasoned that by prescribing bifocals and lessening the focusing effort, the progression can be slowed or halted. We regard the use of bifocals for this purpose as helpful in some cases. The use of contact lenses seems to be more effective. (See Chapter 31, Control of Nearsightedness.)

Prescribing bifocals for children to offset disease or medication is rather rare. Disease may cause a paralysis of the muscles controlling the focusing; the lens may be missing due to a birth defect or cataract surgery. There are some medications which cause blurred reading as a side reaction. If the medication must be used, then bifocals will be needed for the duration of the drug treatment.

Bifocals, then, are not just for old folks, but are of definite value in other cases. As long as there is parental encouragement, children will usually adapt very easily to bifocals.

Part VI

VISION PROBLEMS OF THE AGED

CHAPTER 28

THE VISION OF THE AGING

America is a youth oriented society geared to movement, opportunity, and vitality. For the older person (forced to retire at sixty-five) there is the prospect of uncertainty, economic insecurity, and above all, declining health. It's bad enough to be plagued with arthritis, bursitis, hypertension, neuritis, diabetes, or a score of other maladies, but when vision goes bad, the fear of blindness and losing one's independence becomes a constant worry.

The main causes for such probable loss of sight are cataracts, glaucoma, circulatory problems, and degenerative breakdowns. By far the single biggest cause for potential blindness in older people are cataracts; we have devoted a complete section, Chapter 29 to this topic.

Glaucoma, which is much less common but more dangerous, usually results from poor drainage of the fluid within the eyeball. Since liquid cannot be compressed, too much in the eye will exert pressure on the blood vessels and nerve fibers which gradually choke off the circulation, destroying the nerve fibers and sight. It's usually a slow process which initially reveals itself as a loss of side vision. After a long period of time, if not treated, glaucoma will cause total blindness. There is a rare type of acute glaucoma which strikes suddenly, accompanied by pain, redness, blurry vision, and nausea.

If you have the usual chronic type of glaucoma, you are probably using drops to make the pupil very small and to permit better drainage of the fluid. Some people use oral medication to reduce the amount of fluid in the eye. Those who put drops in the eyes may notice that their vision becomes blurred about a half hour after application. It's something that cannot be avoided. Make sure you aren't involved in any activity such as driving at that time. While drops are effective in retarding glaucoma, with some people they may, unfortunately, contribute to the development of cataracts.

Because very small pupils are induced by the drops, you will need more light for reading. Interestingly, with good light, the constricted pupil may enable you to read without your glasses. Any photography fan will recognize this as the "pinhole camera" effect.

Diabetes, hardening of the arteries, and high blood pressure, may take their toll by causing irreversible damage to the retina. The sight loss can be partial or total depending on the area of the retina involved. On an encouraging note, many types of sight loss can be alleviated with properly designed low vision aids. (See Chapter 39.)

Sometimes a small stroke in the brain can disrupt the control mechanism which points the two eyes together, and you will suddenly see double. This very disturbing situation can last a few days, weeks, months, or for the rest of your life. Special prism glasses can be made which will eliminate or ease the problem.

Even if you manage to avoid these more serious ailments, there are gradual changes on a much more subtle level to live with. For instance, the pupil gets smaller with age and limits the amount of light that can get into the eye. The lens of the eye is less transparent than in youth, which further reduces the light that can reach the retina. The retina itself is less responsive to the light which approaches it. This all adds up to needing more illumination for seeing. Color vision and night vision suffer the most since both require good illumination. Let's put it this way: You men should have little difficulty seeing a woman in a colorful bikini on a bright, sunlit beach, but she might give you some trouble at night. There is not much you can do for these "normal" aging changes, except to use more light when reading and to restrict your night driving.

One of the most frequent complaints from older patients concerns watering and tearing of the eyes. It usually happens when the lids lose some of their muscle tone and no longer rest flush against the eyeball. The moisture which covers the surface of the eye is normally drained into the nose through a thin tube; the opening is located at the inner corner of the lower lid. If this tiny opening is not close against the eye, the tears will simply well up and spill over. When the lid is so loose as to cause profuse tearing, it can be tightened temporarily with tape, or permanently with a simple operation. Another possible reason for watering concerns the tube which is blocked and unable to carry off the tears. A fairly simple procedure is used to unblock it.

A loss of muscle tone can also cause the upper lid to droop. With the exception of the few cases where the lid covers the pupil and interferes with sight, this is mainly a cosmetic problem. The lid can be held up with a fine, flexible metal wire attached to the glasses (ptosis crutch), or lid muscle surgery can be performed.

Seeing black spots, threads, or flies floating around in space is another frequent complaint from our older patients. These complaints are rarely symptoms of a disease, although that possibility must be checked out. Most often they turn out to be tiny specks of solidified material floating around in the fluid part of the eyeball. They may be very annoying, but they cannot be removed. In time they may shift to another part of the eye where they are less noticeable. You also may learn to ignore them. The patient must be reassured that it's not a sign of impending blindness.

Doctors should never be too busy to reassure older people about any particular complaint. Their needs and fears require simple patience and understanding. When the time is taken to carefully explain the condition, it is easier for people to cope with the situation and accept its limitations.

Like most elderly people, you are probably taking medication for one thing or another. You should know that every drug has undesirable side effects; many may affect your vision. For instance, the heart medication, Quinora, can cause double vision, blurred sight, color vision changes, and night blindness. The common nerve drug Valium, may cause blurred and double vision. Your family physician must tell you what side effects you can expect from the prescribed medication.

All in all, the aging process is unkind to health and vision, and requires regular care with understanding and compassion.

CHAPTER 29

CATARACTS, CATARACT SURGERY AND HOW TO COPE

The most common disorder of the eye ultimately leading to loss of sight, is the cataract. Some people have the mistaken idea that a cataract is a growth or film over the eye. It's nothing of the kind. It is a condition wherein the lens of the eye (just behind the colored iris) changes from its clear, transparent state to cloudy and opaque. The experience can be likened to an attempt to see through a steamed-up window.

The clouding is usually quite slow and not the same in both eyes. One eye may even remain totally clear. Unlike a steamed-up window, however, the haze is not evenly distributed and the lens may have opaque areas mixed with clear areas. How much vision you retain depends on the size, location, and density of the cloudy patches.

When we say that the development is slow, we are talking about years. We have often watched patients with small opacities that hardly changed over ten years. By the same token, we have seen a few patients with cataracts that developed in a short period of a few months.

There is no effective treatment to halt or reverse the development of a cataract. We are not entirely sure why people get cataracts as they get older, or why they develop at different rates of time. We suppose that heredity, nutritional, and environmental factors are at work, but we don't know exactly how. Therefore, we have no advice to offer for avoiding them. The only cataracts we can explain are the relatively few which are caused by injuries, high exposure to infra-red rays, and certain medications.

It is quite easy for the optometrist to monitor the progress of your cataract with regular office visits. While this is going on, new glasses will have to be prescribed on a more frequent basis to keep up with your changing vision. If the point is ever reached when a cataract seriously interferes with your sight, it can be removed surgically. But, *don't* rush into surgery until there is little useful vision remaining. We find that most people prefer hazy, but normal vision to the clear, but confusing vision resulting from surgery.

Here's a fairly typical example. Suppose that the right eye has a cataract developing and its sight has decreased. If the left eye also develops a cataract and your overall sight is affected, we would then advise surgery on the right eye. We naturally consider the needs of the individual patient. An eighty-year old, inactive man, who no longer drives, may not be too concerned about 20/60 vision in his better eye, while a fifty-five-year old man could be seriously handicapped long before this stage.

The number of cataract operations performed every year in the United States, is around the 100,000 figure. It is the sixth most common operation, ranking just behind appendectomies. (With ophthalmic surgeons it is number one.) Despite the frequency of the cataract operation, there is no single method followed by all surgeons. The common denominator is a small incision made at the top edge of the cornea. The entire cloudy lens is taken out of the eye, either in one piece or after it has been broken up into small particles with sound waves (phaco-emulsification). Your hospital stay will vary from forty-eight hours to one week.

Sometimes, when there are cataracts of about equal density in both eyes, the surgeon may tell you to have both removed at the same time. This is an offer you should refuse. We have seen too many patients who succumbed to such reasoning, suffer severe visual and emotional problems after the double operation. Because it is difficult to walk around and do normal, everyday tasks, for several months they become totally dependent on other people. We suggest you have only one eye operated on and adjust to that situation before having surgery on the other eye.

(The one exception is in the case of an intraocular lens implant procedure. In this intricate technique, the cloudy lens is replaced with a small plastic disc suspended in front of the iris. There are fewer visual disturbances with this procedure, and both eyes can have the cataracts removed at the same time. Just a few surgeons use this method at present, although the number will probably increase if the complications can be kept to a minimum.)

There are a number of possible combinations. (1) Cataract in one eye, partial cataract in the other eye. (2) Cataract in one eye, no cataract, or only a faint cataract in the other eye. (3) Cataracts in both eyes.

Category number 1 is probably the most common; we'll assume you are in this group. What can you expect after cataract surgery on the one eye? When the cloudy lens has been removed and the healing process is moving along, its sight will be bright, but very blurry; colors will appear exceptionally vivid. The reason for the blurry sight is that the now-missing lens contributed a great deal of refractive power to the normal eye. Without it you are very, very farsighted and need some artificial aid to see.

First you'll be provided with temporary glasses which will give you reasonably good sight in the operated eye, but will blur the unoperated eye. Your sight may vary from day to day because the eye is changing as it heals. You will also have to put up with distortions and an enlarged image from the spectacle lens. After an eight to twelve week healing time, you will be ready for a permanent vision correction.

We recommend being fitted with a contact lens instead of glasses because it creates less visual conflict with the other eye. Why is there less conflict? A spectacle lens of the required strong power enlarges the image about 30%. While

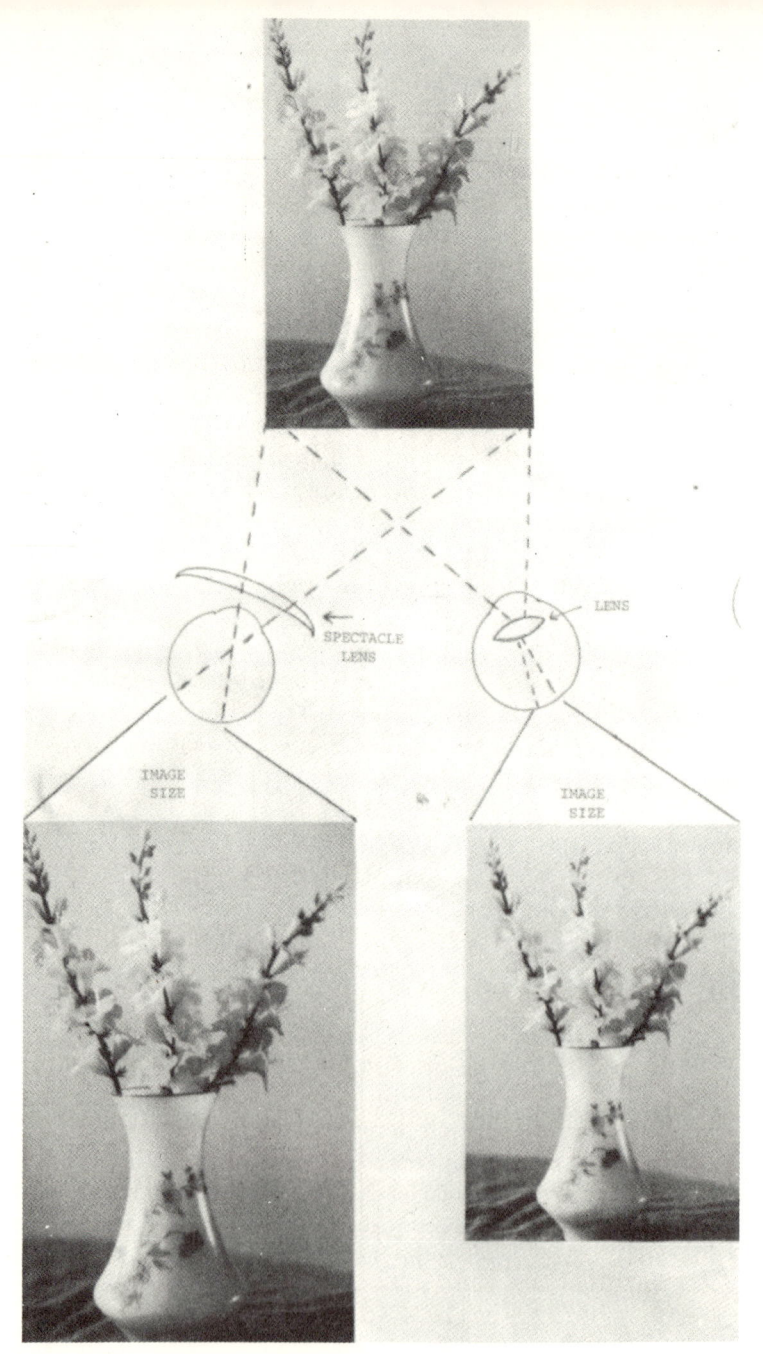

After cataract surgery, a spectacle lens will correct sight but produce magnified image. The brain cannot combine it with normal image as seen by unoperated eye.

you may think it's better to see things larger, it actually makes things worse, because the brain is unable to fuse this enlarged image with the normal size image from the unoperated eye. Intolerable double vision could be the result. With a contact lens, double vision is avoided because the images are about the same size and both eyes can see together.

While the contact lens is a substitute for a thick spectacle lens, it doesn't eliminate glasses entirely. You will have to wear glasses with the contact lens for reading and/or to correct the sight in the unoperated eye.

We know there are circumstances when it is not feasible to use a contact lens (mainly patient fear or inability to handle), and we must resort to glasses. To avoid seeing double you will use either the unoperated *or* operated eye for seeing. If the sight in the *un*operated eye is fairly good, you will continue to use this eye for seeing and the operated eye will be left blurry. If, on the other hand, the sight in the *un*operated eye is very poor, we will prescribe glasses to fully correct the operated eye while blurring the *un*operated one. Although it may be possible to correct your sight to nearly 20/20 this way, you will encounter a few problems. You will have difficulty getting used to the enlarged view of the world and will misjudge distances. The thick spectacle lens will also cause distortions, narrow your field of view, and make walking uncertain. You will gradually adapt to these conditions.

As a result of the cataract operation, most people become more light sensitive and good sunglasses are vital. They should be tinted green or grey and made of glass, because plastic lenses do not filter out any harmful infra-red rays. We realize that glass is heavier, but it's better for sunny, hot, outdoor use. (Plastic sunglasses are fine in cool climate regions without hot summers.) Your regular glasses *should* be made with plastic lenses to ease the weight burden on your nose. For those who are especially light sensitive, a very pale green tint may be helpful.

The fitting and adjustment of cataract glasses on your face is very critical. A small amount of tilt or misalignment will seriously affect the way you see with them. Correctly made and fitted, you should be able to cope quite well. If the cataract then has to be removed from the second eye, your adjustment time will be much shorter.

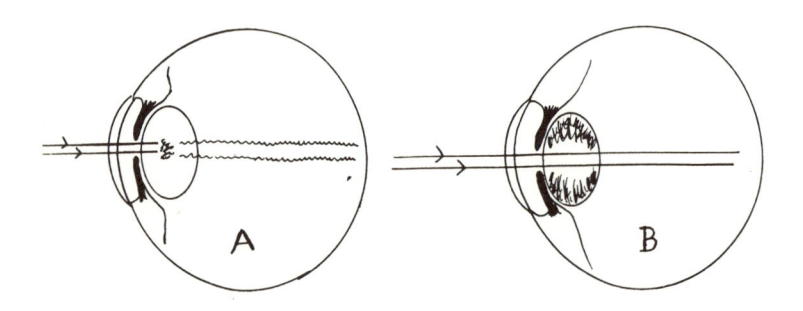

There are many types of cataracts and they will effect vision differently. The tiny cataract in A, being centrally located will cause more sight loss than the much larger peripheral cataract in B.

Part VII

VISUAL THERAPY

CHAPTER 30

WHAT IT IS AND WHEN IT'S INDICATED

Visual therapy refers to any type of treatment procedure geared to correct faults in the visual system. Such a fault may be a conspicuous crossed eye, an unsuspected amblyopic ("lazy") eye, reading difficulties, poor eye coordination, marginal depth perception, etc. The treatment may involve nothing more than spectacles worn as directed, or it may require prism glasses, bifocal glasses, eye patching, light stimulation, or eye exercises.

We use the term "exercise" for lack of a better one, but it should not be thought of as calisthenics. Since the eyes are never at rest, but always moving, the twelve muscles involved get plenty of *physcial* exercise. (Even during sleep there is much eye movement.) In rare cases, when eye movement is restricted by one or more paralyzed muscles, physical exercise will not help. Visual therapy eye exercises are designed to alter and modify the *signals* sent from the control center—the brain.

To make this point clear, we will use the analogy of learning to typewrite. In this practice, you exercise more than your fingers. What you're actually doing is teaching the brain: For every letter you touch on the typewriter, a signal has to be sent to the brain to make the appropriate movement. At first it is necessary to concentrate on each finger, but as you get better, it becomes "automatic." When a typing mistake is made, it's because the brain sent the wrong or an out-of-sequence signal; it is not because one of your fingers is weak, long, or short.

This may surprise you, but in the visual system the wrong signal may be sent *deliberately*, not *accidentally*, to resolve a conflict between clear sight, focusing, and eye movements. The result is a departure from normal vision; the most extreme departure results in a crossed eye. Forget for the moment that a crossed eye is cosmetically unacceptable, or that it deprives the person of depth perception. As far as the brain is concerned, it's a beautiful solution—it avoids the more serious problem of double vision. Furthermore, a crossed eye will not cause disturbing symptoms such as headaches, fatigue, close seeing problems, etc. These symptoms only show up when an eye is *almost* crossed, when the sight from one eye is *almost* supressed, when the ability to focus the two eyes together is *almost* adequate for the task.

The normal, comfortable, three-dimensional vision many of us take for granted, is composed of dozens of complex functions working together in smooth harmony. Like a finely-tuned engine, we're hardly aware of it when all of the systems are working properly. However, if a couple of cylinders stop functioning, the engine will sputter while running; when enough cylinders stop functioning, the engine will come to a halt and you will have to find another mode of transportation. In visual terms, your normal vision will also make compromises with its functions. It may "merely" cause headaches when reading, or more distressingly, cause a crossed, amblyopic eye. Between these two extremes, of course, there are many variations.

To make it more understandable, we have listed the visual functions in increasing order of complexity which are necessary to reach the goal of normal, binocular vision.

1. Each eye must see clearly.
2. Each eye must move easily in all directions.
3. Each eye must see similar images.
4. Both eyes must look at the same object.
5. The brain must fuse the separate images from the two

eyes into one conception.
6. The fusion must produce depth perception.
7. The focusing and eye turning mechanisms of the two eyes must be in balance.
8. There must be ample reserve energy to maintain this balance for long periods of time.

The cross-eyed child, for instance, may only be working with the first few rudimentary functions. It will be a long and difficult road to fully rehabilitate his visual system. The accountant who experiences discomfort and headaches when working, may be struggling with the last two functions only, and his rehabilitation will be much easier. The many possible combinations of visual disorders have varying prospects for full improvement.

Parents get quite upset over a crossed eye, and rightly so. But, they are disturbed for the wrong reason. They view the crossed eye as a cosmetic problem, like buck teeth. If we tackle the eye strictly on the basis of appearance and resort to muscle surgery to straighten it, the eye may "look" straight, but rarely will it "see" straight. The operation by itself will not restore binocular vision. On the other hand, if we can get the two eyes to work together through visual therapy, they both will point straight *and* see straight.

The training for any condition starts with the capacity the visual system has achieved; it gradually works up through the higher levels. Success is greatly dependent upon the motivation of the patient. Persistence during training is a necessity! Although complete success is sometimes not possible, the patient must make the effort, or choose to remain a visual cripple for life.

The visual system carries out five principal programs: (a) seeing clearly; (b) focusing at different distances; (c) moving the eyes to the object of interest; (d) combining the two images into one; and (e) balancing the eye movements with focusing. Visual therapy is made up of various combinations of matching training steps.

There are many procedures and instruments available for each stage of the therapy. Different ones are added as they are needed. We'll describe some of the procedures and instruments in general terms. We have created the following classifications for your convenience, in order to make visual therapy more understandable. In actual practice, however, the categories tend to overlap and several facets may be trained at the same time.

Stimulating an Eye to See

Often an amblyopic eye requires a much stronger corrective lens than its partner. The properly prescribed glasses must be worn at all times. This alone, however, is probably not enough to restore sight. We must find a method to incite that eye to see. The simplest, most traditional, and moderately effective treatment is eye patching. Covering the better eye will force the weaker eye into action and, thus, goad it into seeing. However, since the amblyopic eye sees with an off-center part of the retina, patching the good eye may only reinforce the bad habit and doom the effort. In this case, some doctors will patch the weaker eye to break up this ingrained pattern. Other patching variations for particular cases include screening out the inner half of both eyes or, screening out the center view of the amblyopic eye.

A more dynamic way to stimulate sight is to use some type of light. It can be a flashing light or a very bright light geared to dazzle the center of the retina. Pure light has an advantage: It will not cause conflicts between any visual functions which the brain might be forced to reject.

A method used by some doctors is to put drops into the good eye, paralyzing its focusing, and force the use of the amblyopic eye.

Focusing

Absolute focusing is an automatic reflex, probably activated by those visual cells in the retina which respond to sharp contrast borders. While focusing itself cannot be trained, the speed of the focusing response, as well as its relationship to eye convergence, is possible.

Eye Movements

There are several types of eye movements necessary for good vision. Each eye must be able to track moving objects, change fixation rapidly and accurately, and both eyes must work in unison. Since the tracking ability is based on a feedback mechanism which is dependent on an image being seen with relative clarity, an amblyopic eye is usually poor at smoothly following a target. Treatment involves forcing the eye to pursue rotating targets with, perhaps, a device involving hand/eye coordination. Hand/eye coordination is used in many training procedures; it helps to reinforce the feedback signals. (At times an audible signal is used for reinforcement.) The eye will also be given fixation training so that it can nimbly look from one point to another.

Fusion—Combining 2 Images into 1

It would seem that there is a contradiction in the visual system—there must be two images for the brain to perceive one three-dimensional object. Very closely-matched images for each eye, stimulate specialized brain cells to induce a sense of depth and substance to the physical world. At the same time, the brain cells squelch the two images to keep us from seeing double. Here is the key point: To see in true, full three-dimension, the brain must first be aware of two images.

In the cross-eyed child, the brain ignores (suppresses) the image from the turned eye and, obviously, no fusion is possible. More often, however, it's not that simple. Faulty fusion and intermittent suppression can exist with apparently straight eyes. The first order of business is to make the brain simultaneously aware of an image from *each* eye. The suppression barrier has to be broken down.

Frequently, the suppression and/or turned eye developed as a defense mechanism to avoid consciously seeing two physical objects when there was actually only one. To get around this protective bastion, we initially present large, simple targets to each eye. The brain cannot ignore them because each target is very different—they may differ in form, shape, or only in color. Over a period of weeks or months, the differences in the targets are slowly reduced, brought closer together, made more similar and more complex in design. Finally, when the brain can accept two closely matching targets, three-dimensional vision is kindled. At first the depth perception will be weak and unsteady, but it will be strengthened by continued training.

Balancing Eye Movements With Focusing

If you hold this print about twenty inches away, and slowly bring it back closer, your eyes will do two things: (a) increase focusing power to keep the print clear, and (b) increase convergence to keep the print centered for each eye. A given amount of focusing, accompanied by a matching amount of inward turning of the eyes, are linked together via signals from the brain.

Fortunately, this linkage has a built-in flexibility. This makes it possible to alter the focusing-convergence relationship. The flexibility is a very important factor in maintaining clear, comfortable vision. Without this skill, blurred or double vision may result. The more latitude you have in the linkage, the better off you are. A wide range of flexibility is especially desirable for anyone doing prolonged close work. Without it, you will experience fatigue, headaches, and blurring of print.

Training can expand the flexibility and strengthen the reserve energy needed to maintain it for continuous close work. The procedure involves stimulating the focusing while keeping the convergence quiet, or vice versa. It is done with combinations of prisms, lenses, red-green pictures, mirrors, polarized pictures, etc.

The successful conclusion of a visual therapy program does not always mean you're set for life. Like the baseball player who undergoes spring training then takes batting and fielding practice before each game, it might be necessary to retrain visual skills that have slipped back as time goes by. A change in occupation which requires different visual aptitudes would require such retraining.

The optometrist will, of course, monitor any visual changes during routine office visits. Retraining usually takes much less time and effort than the original sessions.

CHAPTER 31

CONTROL OF NEARSIGHTEDNESS

Nearsightedness, or myopia, has always received more attention than farsightedness. We don't have to look far for the reason—myopia is quite easy to diagnose, even self-diagnose. Myopia simply means that distance sight is poor, but close-up sight is good. Sooner or later the nearsighted youngster becomes aware of a deficiency; his friends can read signs and recognize faces much farther away. Move this child into the classroom and his inability to see the writing on the chalkboard is readily apparent to the teacher. The antiquated wall eye chart used for decades by physicians and schools to test sight, is mainly a screening for myopia. When the child becomes a teen-ager and applies for a driver's license, he will take an eye test mainly concerned with distance sight, and the myope will fail the test.

Since myopia is easy to diagnose, most myopes in the population *are* identified. This is not so with other vision defects. (In the classroom setting, for instance, the farsighted child with a reading problem is not recognized as needing visual care. He is merely considered "slow.")

Because of its stubborn tendency to increase during the growing years, there is a great amount of attention given to myopia. To avoid the steady increases, almost a century of efforts have been made to halt, control, or reverse myopia.

Overall, these efforts have been disappointing. While it is true that we have succeeded with some individuals, the percentage of myopes has been steadily climbing since World

War II. There seems to be little doubt that this "epidemic" is a by-product of our culture.

Recent studies strongly suggest that myopia is directly related to the act of reading, eye focusing, illumination, head and body posture, and nutrition. The single biggest factor is probably related to reading or concentrated close work of any kind. A few years ago, an interesting investigation revealed that Eskimo children, who historically had a low incidence of myopia, showed a remarkable increase once they were required to attend school. A current theory holds that the continuous focusing exertion at near, especially with the head downward (as leaning over a desk), causes an increase in the fluid pressure within the eye. This, in time, enlarges the eyeball. Indeed, the typical myopic eye *is* large and, therefore, out of focus for distance seeing. But, what about the Eskimo children's poor lighting conditions during reading, or their change to a higher sugar intake in diet? As the saying goes: "You pay your money and you take your choice."

At this point, we should consider whether myopia is really a handicap. Think about the nearsighted person who is very much at home with reading and close work, rarely suffering a problem with such tasks. In later life, when the middle-aged farsighted person requires reading glasses, the myope is still blissfully reading without them. The major obstacle for the myope, then, is seeing clearly far away. This can easily be taken care of with glasses or contact lenses. But (and, this is a big *but* for some people), there are psychological and prejudicial handicaps. Ever since Herman Snellen standardized the measurement of visual acuity more than a hundred years ago, the magic of 20/20 sight has made those with a lesser measurement feel inferior. The wearing of glasses was associated with "weak eyes," a silly prejudice which still persists in certain vocational requirements. On balance, the wearing of glasses or contact lenses might be a nuisance at times, but, in small amounts nearsightedness is not a calamity.

We can classify myopia into four categories:
1. Simple.
2. Moderate to high.
3. Degenerative or pathological.
4. Pseudo-myopia.

1. *Simple.* About eight out of ten myopes fit into this group. The nearsightedness starts somewhere between the ages of seven and ten and progresses slowly for the next decade. Small increases in the strength of the glasses are needed every twelve to eighteen months, depending on growth. Spurts in physical growth will produce spurts of increased myopia. The bulk of the changes are over by the age of twenty, unless the person is involved in excessive close work which may push the myopia a little higher. There are no particular damaging retinal problems to be concerned about.

2. *Moderate to High.* About two out of ten myopes are in this group. It starts a little earlier here than with simple myopia, and the changes are more frequent and greater in amount. Spurts in growth produce greater spurts in myopia; it usually levels off somewhat later in life. The higher myopia means a larger eyeball which causes some stretching of the retinal layer at the back of the eye. Because of this development, there is the possibility that ailments such as degeneration or detachment of the retina, will occur later in life.

3. *Degenerative or Pathological.* This rare condition starts at birth or very early in life. The changes are rapid, large in amount and continue into middle age. There are various complications of the retina, frequently leading to sight loss.

4. *Pseudo-myopia.* Unlike the three previous categories, although distance vision is poor, this one is not a true nearsighted condition. The muscles controlling eye focusing at near become "cramped" from excessive close work, and cannot fully relax as they should when the eye looks far away. If this condition continues for a long time, the muscles will maintain the "cramp" and produce the false, or

pseudo-myopia, with variable vision. It can do such a good job of mimicking nearsightedness, that it has even been known to mask farsightedness. With appropriate testing, the doctor should be able to determine the true case.

Compensating for nearsightedness with glasses, is essential. Unfortunately, the glasses do nothing to stop true myopia from increasing. It will increase whether or not you wear your glasses, whether or not you eat carrots, whether or not you practice Yoga, etc.

While we tend to blame reading as the major cause of myopia, obviously not everyone who reads becomes nearsighted. There are other factors we just don't know about yet. Probably heredity plays a big role—some people are just more prone than others. If we ever discover all the reasons for myopia, a true control may be possible. In the meantime, a lively debate is in process over a number of methods which claim to prevent, halt, or reverse myopia. They are:

1. Discontinuing close work entirely.
2. Prescribing glasses with less power than indicated.
3. Wearing bifocal glasses.
4. Wearing contact lenses.
5. Orthokeratology.
6. Visual therapy procedures.
7. Drug therapy.
8. Surgical intervention.

Let's examine and try to evaluate each concept. The first choice, discontinuing close work entirely or even partially, is impractical in our highly technological society. The abstinence from reading might preserve clear distant sight, but the cost would be illiteracy. Also, since we do many things at close range, it's no guarantee for avoiding myopia. For instance, television viewing induces some focusing effort which could plunge the susceptible person into myopia.

Prescribing glasses which are somewhat weaker in power than needed does, in many cases, have a small retarding effect on myopia increase. The amount is very modest, however, and of no great consequence in the overall picture.

Because the theory is elegantly simple, the use of bifocals has many proponents. Assuming that the focusing effort at near causes myopia, bifocals should lessen the focusing effort. Therefore, any increase in myopia would be retarded. In actual practice, it works with some youngsters, but not with others. The habitual reading distance is probably a big factor. Many nearsighted children who are fitted with bifocals will hold the reading material even closer than before. Reading at eight or ten inches virtually negates the effect of the bifocal—focusing is stimulated and myopia progresses on its merry way. Bifocals would be more effective if the reading material was held at sixteen inches, but try to enforce that. If we could get the child to read at eighteen to twenty-two inches without bifocals, it would be most effective. However, the nearsighted child has a "need" to read very close and "enjoys" the large image size. This may very well be the original reason for the myopia.

Clinical experience indicates that giving bifocals indiscriminately to all nearsighted children, is just as wrong as not providing bifocals for those who can benefit from them. The most successful candidate is the child who can be induced to relax his focusing strain. Foremost in this group is the pseudo-myope for whom bifocals, accompanied by visual therapy, is quite effective. For some obscure reason, girls respond better to bifocal application than boys.

The most effective regimen seems to be the wearing of hard contact lenses. It is not unusual for children who did need frequent changes in their glasses, to require no further changes while wearing contacts. The reasons are not clear and the studies reported to date are inconclusive. Some of the factors may be: Corneal curvature changes, pupil size, metabolic changes, alteration in the accommodation-convergence relationship, intra-ocular pressure changes, corneal thickness, relaxation of focusing spasm, molding effect of the contact lens, anterior chamber depth, etc. With so many possibilities, it is difficult to determine which one or which combination holds the myopia in check. On the other hand, some authorities contend that myopia control through wearing contacts is merely an artifact and not yet authenticated.

The new, flexible or soft contact lenses have an as yet unknown effect on myopia reduction. Since the lens is soft, it probably does not have the firm pressure effect on the cornea. We will have to wait a few more years to evaluate the results. Our feeling is that it does slow myopia, but not as well as the hard lenses. In cases of rapidly increasing myopia, for best results, hard contacts should be prescribed at an early age.

A more novel and dramatic use of hard contacts is in the controversial field of orthokeratology. The word derives from "ortho," meaning zero power, and "keratology," referring to the study of the cornea. The proponents of orthokeratology claim to reduce myopia by flattening the cornea with the use of hard contacts. This seemingly compensates for the elongated eyeball so that the image is focused clearly without the need of corrective lenses.

Here's the working principal. The front surface of the cornea is measured with instruments to determine its curvature. Contacts are prescribed to achieve a small flattening effect. As the cornea is reshaped, new lenses are fitted for additional flattening; this cycle is repeated several times. When the reshaping process is completed and 20/20 sight obtained without the need of a correction, the contact lens wearing time is slowly reduced. If the shape of the cornea has been permanently altered, no further correction is necessary. However, for most people the cornea will gradually resume its former curvature and vision will decline. At this stage, "retainer" lenses are fitted to hold the shape of the cornea in check. They are the final lenses (hopefully) which will be needed. To maintain their good vision, some people have to wear the retainer lenses six to eight hours a day, some wear them while sleeping (!), some wear them a few hours every two or three days, and a few, very rare individuals, can get by with one wearing every couple of months.

The length of the orthokeratology procedure is anywhere from eighteen months to three years. With some people it is possible to obtain satisfactory results if the myopia correction is low or moderate; other people do not respond well at all. For very nearsighted individuals, the best that can be hoped for is a reduction in the power of the correcting lenses. Therefore, for high myopes, we consider orthokeratology of dubious value. There's too much trouble and expense involved. Even with the low myope, we urge great caution since the actual mechanism and the long range effects are unknown. It will be many years before we can be certain if orthokeratology is a panacea, a useful tool in some cases, or merely another failure in the battle against myopia.

The success of visual therapy in controlling myopia is very difficult to assess. We know with proper training, it is possible to relieve the stress of focusing and convergence while reading. It also works well in cases of pseudo-myopia and is successful in bringing about focusing relaxation. However, a total program of therapy to halt myopia is another matter. The idea of a six, seven, or eight-year old following a strict therapy routine, is hard to swallow. The doctors who claim to have achieved control of nearsightedness by using certain therapy instruments, apparently, have very obedient young patients or a remarkable facility to command compliance. We cannot envision a high success ratio.

The use of drug therapy to control myopia relies on the principal of avoiding all focusing at near. Drugs are instilled into the eyes to paralyze the focusing mechanism for weeks and months at a time. The method has little to recommend it as it interferes with the development of the child's visual patterns.

The value of proper nutrition can be guessed at, but proof is hard to come by. Going back for a moment to the earlier cited Eskimo children, you will recall that the increased incidence of myopia was apparently caused by intensified reading and close work. Or was it the change in their habitual eating patterns, or their poor illumination? When civilization altered the Eskimo's life style, it brought with it processed and "junk" foods commonly devoured by our kids. Almost everything we eat has refined sugar and loads of additives. The dangers inherent in such diets are now being discovered. The eye is an extension of the brain, and nervous tissue is very susceptible to ingested chemicals. Some food additives found in hot dogs, among other items, have been implicated in causing hyperactivity and, in certain children, learning problems. It is safe to suggest that sugar-laden breakfast cereals, soft drinks and candy be drastically reduced from the diet. Even if it doesn't control myopia, the general health of the child (and adult) will benefit.

Surgical intervention to reduce or control myopia is a desperate, last resort—it is very risky. Few surgeons will even consider using the exotic surgical techniques. These methods should be avoided; there is a great danger that sight can be completely lost from inflammation, degeneration or infection.

Prevention and control of myopia will continue to be debated, and hopefully, the results will bring us some further solutions. We can anticipate a time in the future when the emphasis will be on preventing the onset of myopia, or, if unavoidable, keeping the amount to a minimum. Someday, your child may come home exitedly from the eye doctor: "Look ma, my myopia only increased a quarter of a diopter this checkup!"

Part VIII

COMMON EYE DISEASES AND DISORDERS

CHAPTER 32

EXTERNAL PARTS

I. LIDS.

1. *Blepharitis:* Inflammation of the lid margin with redness and swelling. It may be associated with allergies and dandruff scales. In the mild form there is a crusting of the lash bases. Some lashes fall out, but grow back. Severe blepharitis (ulcerative) affects the lash follicles; there is a permanent loss of lashes with distortion of the lid margin.

2. *External hordeolum* or *sty:* Infection of a hair follicle (similar to a boil). It begins with a general swelling and pain of the lid, then localizes into a red area with a yellowish center at the lid margin. Breaks open to discharge pus and heals readily.

3. *Chalazion:* Chronic, sometimes inflammatory enlargement of one of the lid glands. Appears as a bump or swelling which slowly increases in size. There is usually no pain.

4. *Internal hordeolum* or *sty:* Infection of a gland on the underside of the lid.

5. *Ptosis:* Drooping of the upper lid. It may be a congenital condition due to a paralysis of the lid muscles or a neurological disorder. Mostly, however, it is seen in older people when there is a loss of muscle tone.

6. *Entropion:* The margin of the lid turns inward causing the lashes to rub and irritate the cornea. Occurs most often in older people or following an injury or a burn.

7. *Ectropian:* The margin of the lid turns outward causing excessive tearing as well as itching and burning of the exposed inner lid. Occurs usually in older people from loss of muscle tone.

8. *Cysts and Tumors:*
   (a) *Xanthelasma:* Flat, yellowish, fatty growth on the surface of the lids, especially near the inner corner. It causes no problem unless there are many large ones which are cosmetically unacceptable.
   (b) *Cyst of gland of Moll:* Small, transparent, watery cyst at the lid margin.
   (c) *Nevus:* Benign tumor which may be pigmented. It is frequently present from birth, but goes unnoticed until it begins to enlarge later in life. In only very rare cases does it become malignant.
   (d) *Malignant tumors:* Can involve any of the cell layers of the lids. The majority occur on the lower lid.

9. *Trachoma:* A viral infection of the inside lid. It gives a granular, cobblestone appearance. It is uncommon in the U.S., but is a major cause of blindness in some parts of the world.

10. *Trichiasis:* One or more lashes grow inward and cause irritation by rubbing the cornea.

11. *Dacryocystitis:* Infection of the tear drainage sac located near the inner corner of the eye. Mild cases exhibit some redness and slight swelling. Severe cases cause pain and obvious swelling.

II. CONJUNCTIVA. Thin transparent membrane covering

the inner surface of the lid and the surface (white) of the eye.

1. *Conjunctivitis:* The common "red eye" or "pink eye."

(a) *Allergic:* The main symptom is itching accompanied by redness. In some cases the inside surface of the upper lid becomes involved with cobblestone-shaped elevations and a thick secretion.

(b) *Infectious (bacterial):* The symptoms are itching, tearing, sensitivity to light and a gritty sensation. The condition can be acute or drag on as a mild, chronic infection. The lids may be stuck together from the discharge, especially when awakening in the morning.

(c) *Infectious (viral):* The symptoms are similar to the bacterial type, but frequently the cornea becomes involved with serious consequences.

2. *Hemorrhage:* A spontaneous hemorrhage can occur on the white of the eye giving a bright, blood-red appearance. Sometimes it is caused by coughing, sneezing, or rubbing the eyes too hard.

3. *Pinguecula:* A small, yellowish elevation on the white of the eye, usually on the nasal side. It becomes more noticeable with age, but is harmless.

4. *Pterygium:* A triangular shaped elevated, vascular tissue on the white of the eye. It is harmless unless it grows across the cornea and blocks sight.

III. CORNEA. The clear cover over the colored part of the eye.

1. *Arcus senilis:* A grey or whitish ring (or part of a ring) around the edge of the cornea. Very common with aging and quite harmless.

2. *Keratitis:* An inflammation of the cornea.

(a) *Superficial:* The infection starts at the surface from an outside source. Depending on the infecting agent, various ulcerations can occur leaving opaque scars after healing.

(b) *Deep:* Transmitted via the blood stream and usually confined to inner layers. The most common type is caused by congenital syphillis and will show up in children and teen-agers.

3. *Keratoconous:* The central area of the cornea becomes thin and bulges forward into a conical shape. Vision is always affected.

4. *Abrasion:* A breakdown of the surface layer of the cornea accompanied by pain, tearing and light sensitivity. Injury or contact lens wear are usually the causes.

5. *Vascularization:* The blood vessels invade the cornea (which is usually devoid of any vessels). It can be caused by disease, inflammation or injury.

6. *Ulceration:* Erosion of the corneal surface caused by bacteria, fungus or virus. It always causes scarring and in extreme cases may perforate through the entire cornea.

IV. SCLERA. The tough, white outer layer of the eyeball.

1. *Episcleritis:* Inflammation of the loose connective tissue of the sclera. It looks very much like conjunctivitis, except that it is usually restricted to a small area, and is a deep red or purple color.

2. *Staphyloma:* A small pigmented bulge in the white of the eye caused by a thinning of the sclera.

CHAPTER 33

INTERNAL PARTS

I. IRIS. A thin, pigmented membrane lying in front of the lens. The pupil is the central opening. The color of the eye is actually the color of the iris.

1. *Iritis:* Inflammation of the iris and ciliary body (to which the iris is anchored) causes pain, extreme light sensitivity, redness and a constricted or irregularly shaped pupil.

2. *Heterochromia:* The iris of one eye is different in color than the iris of the other eye. It is usually congenital and harmless. A recent color change is associated with iritis.

3. *Synechiae:* The iris adheres to the lens of the eye producing pain and an irregularly shaped pupil. It usually follows iritis. The iris may sometimes adhere to the back of the cornea following an injury or eye surgery.

4. *Coloboma:* A congenital defect wherein part of the iris is missing. It can also occur after an injury or eye surgery.

5. *Tumors and cysts:* Can develop in the iris, ranging from harmless to highly malignant.

6. *Iridodonesis:* Tremulous iris due to a displaced or missing lens.

II. LENS. Transparent, semi-elastic structure which can change shape to focus at different seeing distances.

   1. *Subluxated lens:* The lens is shifted out of its normal position, usually down. It may be congenital or resulting from an injury. Vision is affected depending on the degree of displacement.

   2. *Cataract:* The lens of the eye becomes cloudy. It is not a growth or film, but a gradual transformation of transparent lens fibers becoming opaque. The most common type is the "senile," associated with aging. The density and location of the opacities will determine the sight loss.

III. VITREOUS. The clear, jelly-like material which fills the inside of the eye behind the lens.

   1. *Muscae volintantes* or *Floaters:* Small, solidified particles floating in the vitreous which are seen as spots, threads or specks when looking at a bright background. Harmless, but annoying when in the line of sight.

IV. RETINA. The thin nerve layer covering the inside back of the eye where light is absorbed and converted into electrical signals for sight. Since the retina is profusely supplied with surface blood vessels, general vascular changes can be seen in the eyes.

   1. *Arteriosclerosis:* The arterial walls become thickened, restricting the blood flow. As the condition worsens, small hemorrhages may occur. A possible serious consequence is an obstruction of a main artery or vein.

   2. *Hypertensive retinopathy:* General high blood pressure will, of course, involve the retinal vessels. Besides arteriosclerosis, there may be edema, exudates, and hemorrhages. The site and extent of retinal damage will determine the sight loss.

3. *Diabetic retinopathy:* Long-standing diabetes will cause engorgement of the veins and the formation of aneurisms. The resulting hemorrhages and exudates will interfere with vision. It is a leading cause of visual impairment.

4. *Arterial/Venous occlusion:*
   (a) An obstruction of the central retinal artery or a principal branch, will cause loss of vision either totally (main artery), or in the area supplied by the branch.
   (b) An obstruction in a major vein causes massive hemorrhages and sight impairment. As the hemorrhage is slowly absorbed, there is a gradual sight improvement.

5. *Papillitis:* Inflammation of the optic nerve disc.

6. *Papilledema:* The optic nerve disc becomes swollen. The usual cause is an increase in the intracranial pressure and interference with venous circulation of the eye.

7. *Retinitis Pigmentosa:* Degeneration of the retina and gradual loss of vision. Early symptom of this hereditary disease is night blindness.

8. *Retinal degeneration:* Disturbances in the vascular system will usually lead to degenerative changes. It affects mostly older people with vision gradually being reduced.

9. *Macular degeneration:* Disturbances in the central retinal area (macula), result in sight loss.

10. *Choroiditis:* Inflammation of the choroid which affects the overlying retina. It is caused by a systemic disease which is often difficult to identify. The inflammatory lesions can be at the extreme side with little visual disturbance, or near the macula, with decided sight loss. The inflammation slowly subsides, but repeated attacks are common.

11. *Tumors:* May be malignant or benign. An early symptom may be sight loss due to a retinal detachment.

12. *Retinal detachment:* Any break or tear in the retina can be followed by detachment from the underlying choroid. Possible causes may be a congenital condition, injury, disease, malignant myopia.

V. OPTIC NERVE. The collection of some million individual nerve fibers connecting the eye to the brain.

1. *Optic atrophy:* The optic nerve fibers are destroyed as a result of disease, injury or pressure directly on the nerve. Portions of the central and/or side vision are lost.

2. *Toxic amblyopia:* Loss of central vision due to chronic poisoning, usually tobacco or alcohol.

3. *Retrobulbar neuritis:* Inflammation of the optic nerve which is usually accompanied by painful eye movements and loss of central vision.

4. *Tumors:* Any tumors along the nerve pathway will cause a gradual loss of vision, often accompanied by exophthalmos.

VI. ORBIT. The eye is enclosed in a bony vault surrounded with fatty tissue.

1. *Inflammation:* Bacterial infection of the tissue and fat around the eye.

2. *Tumors:* A variety of tumors can occur. The most obvious symptoms are a bulging eye and double vision.

3. *Exophthalmos:* Bulging eyes. When both eyes are involved, the condition is caused by an over-active thyroid. Only one eye bulging is caused by a tumor, inflammation or vascular condition.

4. *Enophthalmos:* The appearance of a sunken eyeball. It usually follows an injury or occurs in older people when some of the fatty tissue is absorbed.

VII. GLAUCOMA. Increase in the fluid pressure within the eye causes interference with the blood supply and damage to the sensitive retinal nerves. There is a progressive loss of sight beginning peripherally.

1. *Chronic:* About 90% of glaucoma is in this category. It has a slow course (many years) without pain and few symptoms in the early stages. Colored halos around lights may be seen on occasion.

2. *Acute:* This accounts for about 5% of glaucoma. There is a sudden attack of blurred sight, pain, nausea, red eye and an enlarged immobilized pupil.

Part IX

THE PARTIALLY SIGHTED

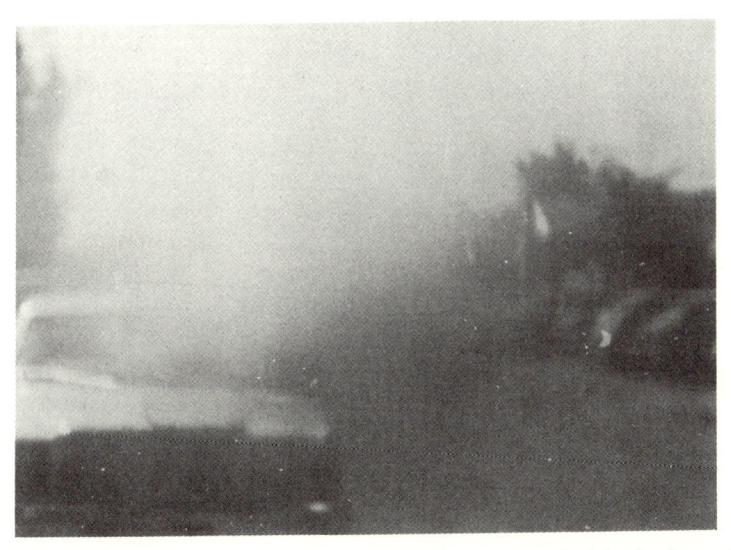

This is the way a street scene would look to an eye with the loss of central vision.

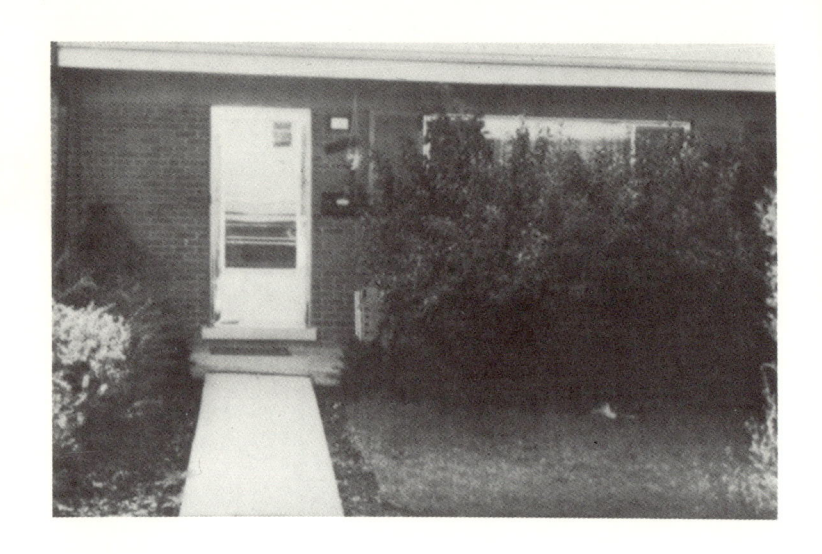

The total field of view as seen by a normal eye. (Above) The same view as seen by an eye with some peripheral field losses. (Below)

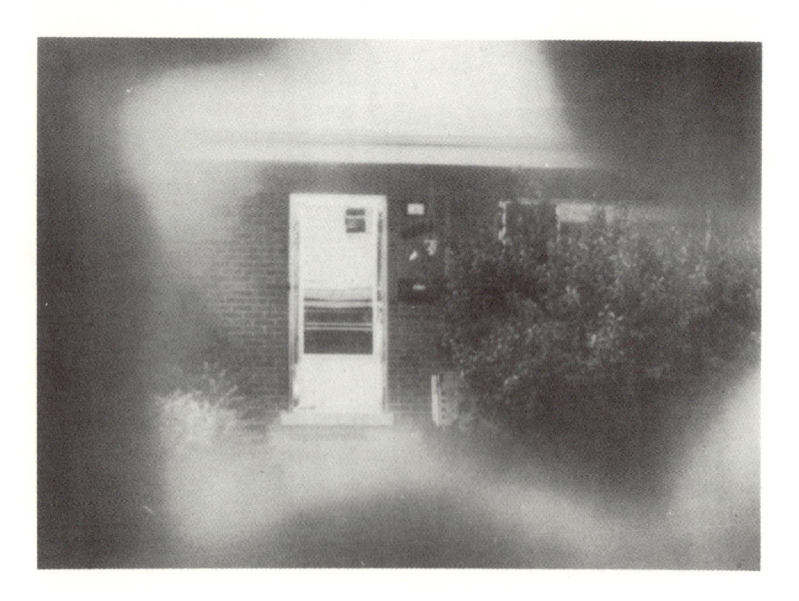

CHAPTER 34

WHAT IT IS AND WHO CAN BE HELPED

Anyone who has a significant sight impairment and cannot see clearly with regular glasses, is considered to be partially sighted. Anyone who has a blind area in the visual field which hinders or prevents walking around with comfort, is also considered to be partially sighted.

The term "partially sighted" is rather imprecise; it covers a wide range of vision conditions. It can mean relatively good sight, with a best corrected acuity of approximately 20/50; it can mean legal blindness (less than 20/200); it can mean good straight ahead sight with restricted side vision; it can mean good side vision with poor straight ahead sight; it can mean any combination of the above.

Regardless of the category, degree of sight loss, or age, improvement is usually possible. If a doctor has told you that nothing more can be done, the odds are four to one the doctor is wrong. A very disquieting statement, but all too true. Most ophthalmologists know little about devising optical systems to make maximum use of the available sight. They will treat the disease causing the sight loss, then let the afflicted patient live with the handicap. This is quite regrettable. Ideally, there should be a joint effort by an ophthalmologist treating the disease, and an optometric low vision specialist to recoup and restore as much vision as possible.

It is difficult for the sighted person to imagine what it's like to live at the edge of blindness. Most people have the notion that blindness can be likened to the experience of darkness when the eyes are shut. Usually, it's not so. Legal blindness refers to a person whose corrected sight in the *better* eye is 20/200 or less, or when the field of view in the *better* eye is 20 degrees or less. With 20/200 you'd be hard pressed to either recognize faces or read anything but newspaper headlines. The restriction of a 20 degree field is like looking through a tube, rendering it awkward and difficult to walk around. (The normal field is seven to eight times larger.)

The legal definition for blindness was established in the 1930s; "corrected" means that the afflicted person wears conventional eyeglasses. It does not take into account the many new advances and aids that can assist the partially-sighted persons, nor does it reveal the true ability of the patient to function in the world.

The partially-sighted person should not meekly accept this handicap until he or she has consulted an optometrist who specializes in low vision care. One of us (Herb Solomon), has been involved in low vision work for many years and is convinced that eight out of ten people can be helped.

This does not necessarily mean that improvement will reach 20/20, but it could be the difference between seeing a grandchild's face in blurry outline or seeing the freckles on it; between struggling with a newspaper headline or reading the story; between walking with hesitation, holding a white cane or walking without assistance on your own.

The number of *totally* blind people in this country is about 500,000. The number of partially-sighted people is much greater, between 2,500,000 to 5,000,000. If nothing is done to keep them functioning visually, many of these people may despondently slip into the ranks of the blind.

Some people, of course, have a better chance of being helped than others. It depends on the type of vision loss and personal temperament. Can you be helped? If you can answer "yes" to at least five of the following questions, you are an excellent prospect:

1. Do you have a strong desire to be self-sufficient, to do things without the help of others?
2. Are you willing to try new things which may improve your sight?
3. Has your sight remained essentially the same during the past two years?
4. Can you get around fairly easily when alone in an unfamiliar place?
5. Can you recognize faces at four or more feet?
6. Can you read street signs or house numbers at five or more feet?
7. Are you light sensitive? Can you see better with less light?
8. Do you have fairly good color vision and do you enjoy color TV?
9. Can you read newspaper headlines or smaller print?
10. Can you read large print with a magnifying lens?

If this test indicates that you can be helped, contact your family optometrist. He or she can refer you to a low vision specialist.

A comprehensive low vision examination includes many exhaustive tests as well as a trial application of optical aids suited to your specific visual requirements. It will take a total of four to eight hours spread over a few weeks. At the end of that time, you will have a good idea of how much sight improvement you can expect.

CHAPTER 35

THE VISUALLY-IMPAIRED CHILD

Discovering that your child has a serious visual problem bordering on blindness is a devastating experience. Not counting eye injuries, such problems are usually brought on by congenital conditions or hereditary defects. The congenital cases are frequently caused by the use of drugs or a viral infection which occurred during pregnancy. We are not referring to illicit drugs, particularly, but medication legally prescribed by physicians. One need only remember back a few years to the havoc created by Thalidomyde, a drug which was legal at the time.

The most common conditions causing sight impairment in children are: Albinism (lack of pigment), cataracts, retrolental fibroplasia, aniridia (lack of iris), scarring of the cornea, nystagmus (rapid, oscillating eye movements), and degenerative myopia.

Can this child lead a reasonably normal life? Is regular schooling possible? The answer to each question is a qualified "yes." If the child has a stable, congenital condition, he can be helped rather easily to see better and have a fairly normal life. Children have a knack for adjusting to situations, and readily learn to use optical aids. They will even adopt ways of seeing which may seem strange to you. For instance, it is not unusual for a child with poor distant sight to be able to read small print held a few inches away. It is almost impossible for an adult to read that close. The explanation rests with the large amount of focusing power available to the young eye. By taking advantage of it, the child may get along quite well in school, using only telescopic spectacles to see the chalkboard.

Schools across the country handle the partially-sighted child in different ways. Some will lump them all together in classes for the visually handicapped; others will base the separation on the degree of attainable functional vision. The latter, of course, is the preferred method. We urge each school district to obtain the services of an optometric low vision specialist to evaluate each child individually. With additonal help from resource teachers, it will usually be possible for the child to attend regular classes.

In the classroom, the child's seating must be carefully chosen. It is not just a matter of being close to the chalkboard, though that may be necessary, but also the partially-sighted child must be in a seat which is compatible with his individual lighting requirements. Some require strong illumination, others need low levels. For example, an albino child may have to be shielded from sunlight streaming in through the window, and may have to wear tinted lenses, side shields, or even a visor to protect him from overhead light. Another child may need a good desk lamp to light up his reading material. Reflections from shiny surfaces, only mildly annoying to a normal child, can be a serious visual irritant to the partially-sighted child.

Some of these youngsters will require writing guides, special pencils and heavily lined notebook paper. It will usually take them a little longer to complete their assignment, and teachers should provide the extra time. Participation in most school activities can be encouraged, but if the child has only one usable eye, body contact sports are to be avoided.

If you keep in mind that good sight is only one part of the complex system we call vision, you will realize that, while very important, correcting the sight is not enough. We advocate that the child be given visual therapy for better eye movements, hand eye coordination, an established pattern for the two eyes to work together, etc. Some of this therapy can be done in the school, closely supervised by the teacher and monitored by the optometrist.

So far we've been discussing the school-age child. What about the younger child? Depending on the child's ability to understand their use, optical aids for sight improvement can be prescribed. The optometrist will guide the parents in setting up a visual development program for the child. Just as you must walk to develop the leg muscles, the eye must see to learn to see. If the problem is juvenile cataracts, for example, the cataracts must be removed at the earliest possible time so that the system can learn to see. After a successful operation, glasses or contact lenses can improve the sight dramatically.

Contact lenses can, and are, prescribed for very young children. The contacts have to be inserted and removed by an adult, but the lenses are quite safe when carefully fitted. Other situations which lend themselves beautifully to contacts are cases of scarred or irregular corneas, degenerative myopia, and when very strong corrections are needed.

Contact lenses are only one example of novel ways to enable your child to see. We find that some parents are hesitant to allow the fitting of unusual devices because of some vague feeling that it may "use up" the child's vision. This myth belongs in the same wastebasket as the belief that you can "use up" your brain by learning or remembering too much. A few parents veto unusual looking optical aids because it makes the child look different from other children. We can sympathize with this feeling, but depriving the child of vision is too much of a penalty to pay. Marvelous things are possible when you open your mind and allow your child to see. If you transmit a feeling of confidence, your child will adapt to almost any situation.

CHAPTER 36

EDUCATIONAL AND VOCATIONAL OUTLOOK

The education of the partially-sighted teen-ager should be geared to the vocational possibilities that will be open to him or her. It's a good idea to get advice from the optometrist, an opthalmologist, educator, vocational guidance counselor, etc. Keep in mind that visually handicapped people are often met with the same prejudices in obtaining employment as totally blind people.

Students with moderate visual handicaps, which we can define by rule of thumb as poor distance vision, but adequate near vision, usually have little difficulty completing high school. As with normally-sighted students, success with schoolwork as well as the ability to enter college, depends on intelligence, motivation, interest, and aptitudes. If the near vision is good enough to read textbook print, these students, with additional help as needed from special resource teachers, can attend regular classes. (Of course, distance vision will have to be corrected with telescopic aids.) The optometrist should work closely with the teachers to determine if the visual needs are being met. For example, if near seeing becomes troublesome in the upper grades, reading glasses may be needed.

There is one visual area which is usually very blurry for the partially sighted and often neglected—the intermediate range from about ten inches to three feet. This is the range where such things as typing, laboratory experiments in chemistry and physics, and shop work are done. If at all practical, the student may try to "poke his nose" to within a few inches to see the work, otherwise he will just give up and avoid the task. The alert low vision specialist will prescribe special visual aids such as near telescopes, hand magnifiers and adjustable reading stands to cope with these situations. When this is done, a new dimension is opened for the student.

It is much easier to plan the educational and vocational future for the teen-ager with a stable, moderate visual handicap. The stable condition assures fewer changes in low vision aids, and the moderate condition does not severely limit the choice of job opportunities. The only real limitation would be work requiring critical distance seeing, i.e., driving a bus, operating a crane, etc. On the other hand, many blue-collar and most white-collar jobs are quite suitable. The newspaper want-ads show that about 80% can be managed successfully (provided hiring prejudices are overcome).

If the visual impairment is severe or rapidly worsening, finishing high school and college becomes an arduous task. We have to resort to stronger, hence more limiting visual aids (large print books, projection devices) and obtain the services of trained readers. Besides the elimination of jobs requiring critical distance seeing, when thinking about a vocation, there is the limitation imposed by how much vision improvement is possible at near. Most blue-collar and many white-collar jobs have to be passed up, but some can be handled. For instance, becoming a bank teller would be impractical, but becoming a credit analyst in that same bank would be appropriate.

If the prognosis is for nearly total blindness, braille should be learned and preparations made for jobs relying on hearing and touch.

CHAPTER 37

RECENT SIGHT LOSS

For an adult, a recent and rapid loss of sight is usually accompanied by severe emotional distress. It matters little if the sight loss has been caused by disease or injury; a person's entire life is disrupted. The immediate reaction is fear—fear of not being able to carry on in the usual way, of losing a job, of being a financial burden on the family, of becoming dependent on others. Simple, everyday tasks such as shaving, putting on cosmetics, reading food labels, and even seeing the food on a dinner plate become very difficult and frustrating. Is it any wonder that depression sets in? In this despondent state, the person will seek miracle cures to restore his or her sight. ("Just make the glasses a little stronger, Doc.") The harsh reality is that there is no such cure.

Going from doctor to doctor in search of a miraculous vision restoration, is in itself a strong symptom that you are not ready for realistic help. It often takes several years of psychological soul searching to admit that you will never again see the way you used to, that arduous compromises and adjustments will have to be made. Once you do realize it, however, you are ready for sophisticated low vision care.

While you are still struggling with the shock of the sight loss, lean on the optometric low vision specialist for help. You may not be ready for full application of the many marvelous devices available, but the optometrist can provide you with temporary optical and non-optical aids. You can also be apprised of agencies established for your benefit, be referred for the proper medical services, psychological or social counseling.

CHAPTER 38

THE PARTIALLY SIGHTED AS A DRIVER

Incredible as it sounds, it's possible to be legally blind and receive a driver's license (lawfully) in at least twenty states. It isn't done with sleight of hand, but with a telescopic viewing system and/or telescopic glasses. Some states will grant a license if you can demonstrate 20/70 sight; some require 20/50 or 20/40. However, merely being able to see 20/70, 20/40, or even 20/20, does not make someone a safe driver. There are visual and mobility skills which are just as indispensable as sight. Before undertaking the lengthy process leading to obtaining a driver's license for a partially-sighted person, we require the following:

1. A stable visual condition which will not change in the near future.
2. Adequate color vision to clearly distinguish red from green traffic signals.
3. Unrestricted eye movements and the ability to look quickly from one object to another.
4. Normal and unrestricted head movements.
5. A field of view encompassing about 130 degrees with each eye, and no significant blind or missing areas.

To understand the significance of a wide field of view when driving, imagine your car windows steamed up except for one small, clear area directly ahead of you. No matter how well you can see through that clear spot, it obviously would be very dangerous to drive. Normal peripheral vision extends about 90 degrees outward from each eye; we will not accept less than 70 degrees. Since only fifteen states test the field of vision, it's up to the optometrist to determine if the partially-sighted person meets the minimum requirements.

The preferred way to improve sight for driving is with the telescopic viewing system (contact lenses plus glasses). Once you have adapted to this set-up, you should be able to drive fairly easily. The hitch for many partially-sighted persons is that this system only works well with moderate sight losses. For those needing greater sight improvements, we resort to bioptic telescopes. It takes patience, practice, and time (two to four months) to reach the point where you can use these glasses "automatically." You have to get used to such things as objects appearing larger, an altered sense of distance and depth, and objects popping in and out of the field of view with your eye movements. Before allowing you to take the driving test, the low vision specialist will work closely with the driving instructor to make sure of your proficiency under traffic conditions.

At the present time, Dr. Solomon has forty patients who have obtained driver's licenses and are safely handling automobiles while wearing sophisticated telescopic aids and systems.

For many partially sighted persons, driving an auto is at the bottom of their list of priorities. But, if it's important, it may be possible to help you.

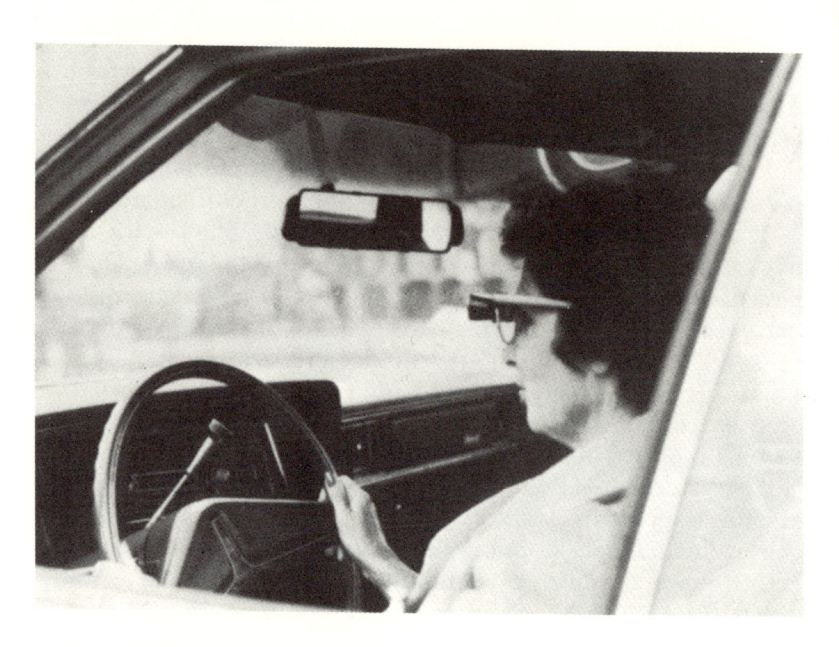

With the use of bioptic telescopes such as these, many partially sighted persons are able to drive an auto.

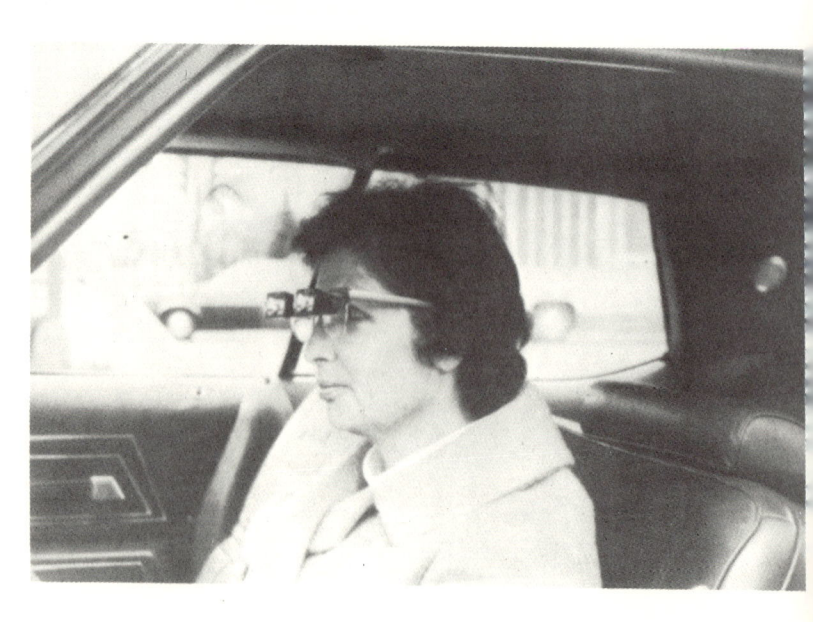

CHAPTER 39

OPTICAL AND NON-OPTICAL AIDS TO HELP YOU SEE

Very often the partially-sighted person is left on his own to find a better way to see. He may drift into a department store and try the use of a hand magnifier; a well-meaning friend or relative may present him with one as a gift. Though the basic idea is sound and he may derive some benefits from the magnifier, they will be limited because: (a) the magnifiers generally available on the retail market are of low power; (b) he may not know how to use it effectively; (c) it will only be useful for a particular task; or (d) if it doesn't work, he will reject all magnifiers.

Normally, the human eye can see across a wide range of distances. For the partially-sighted person this ability is sharply curtailed. Consequently, a number of different aids are needed for seeing at different distances. It all depends on the amount of visual loss, what precisely needs to be seen and how far away it is.

Let's illustrate this concept with Mrs. L., a sixty-year old woman with only 10% vision left after retinal degeneration. For television and movies she uses tiny telescopes fused to her glasses. For cooking and doing housework within a distance of a few feet, she uses near bioptic telescopes and a hand magnifier. Last, for reading or close detail work, she uses very strong reading glasses with intense lighting. To the sighted person, this multiplicity of aids might seem cumbersome and complicated. For Mrs. L., blind for all practical purposes without them, they represent access to the sighted

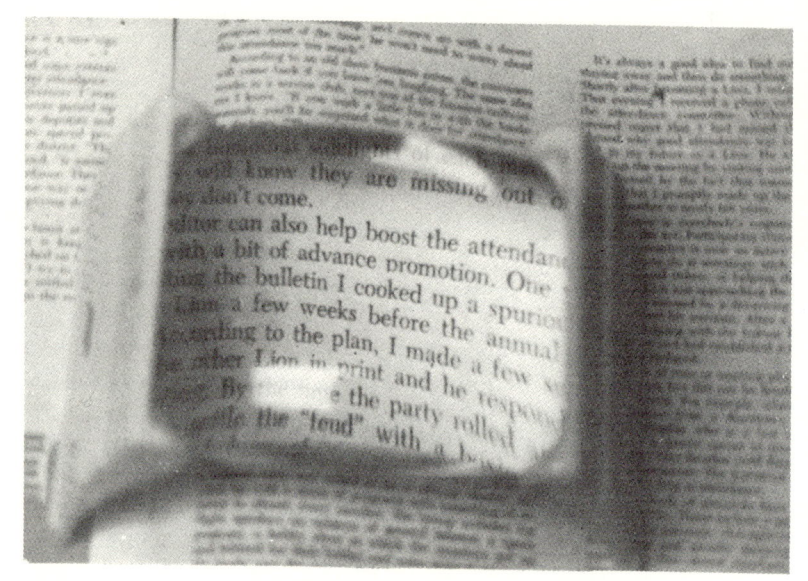

A stand magnifier useful for reading.

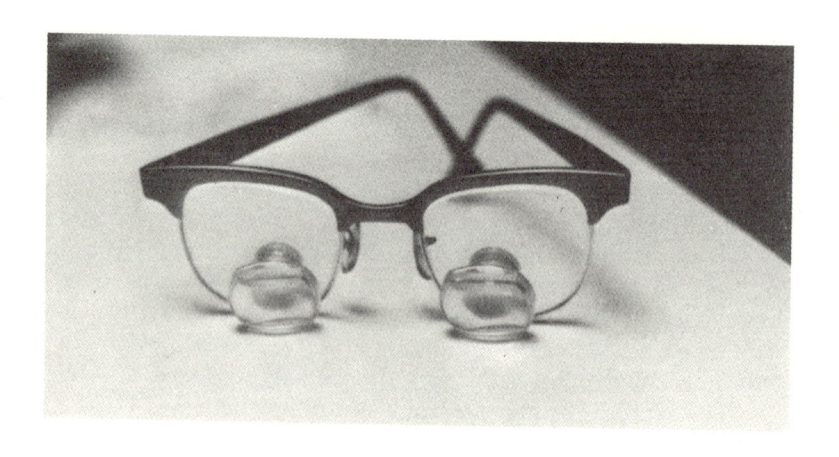

Glasses fitted with near telescopes for reading, sewing, etc.

world and she is delighted. Of course, not all partially-sighted patients require the same help Mrs. L. has been given. The point is, however, the various visual needs of the individual must be evaluated and satisfied, if possible.

The underlying theory for improving sight is to make the object larger and bolder, hence easier to recognize. How can this be accomplished? The simplest way is to actually enlarge the size of the object. In this category are non-optical aids such as large print books, magazines, and newspapers; large numbers on telephone dials; large eyes in needles, etc. It is impractical to rely entirely on this solution; the material is often not available.

Another way to enlarge what you want to see is by relative size magnification. This simply means that the closer you get to an object, the larger it appears. For instance, newspaper print which the partially-sighted person cannot read at sixteen inches, might well be legible at eight inches because it is relatively twice as large; at four inches it appears four times as large. The print is not actually any larger, but by bringing it closer, the image on the retina is enlarged. That leaves only one complication—the eye must be able to focus at a very close distance. Partially-sighted children have little problem since at their age they have great focusing ability. The older person is not as fortunate because focusing ability decreases with age. The optometrist overcomes this by prescribing optical aids to make things clear at the very close viewing distance. It can be done with special microscopic glasses, magnifiers, or loupes attached to glasses.

That takes care of near seeing, but what about looking at television or movies? The only solution is a device which has the ability to enlarge distant objects, namely, a telescope. Some partially-sighted persons who require very high magnification in order to see, actually watch television through binoculars (two telescopes side by side). As you can imagine, it becomes very fatiguing and annoying to hold them still; slight movements cause the image to waver and jump.

A much more convenient method is to use telescopic

clip-ons over spectacles. Though the view through them is rather narrow, it's sufficiently wide to see a TV screen at about ten feet. However, the telescopic clip-ons are useless for walking around.

The most functional and convenient system which *does* permit walking, is a tiny telescope permanently attached to the upper part of the spectacles. Compact and light in weight, it has enough power and an adequate field of view to be useful for extended periods of time. This design is called a bioptic telescope and works like an upside-down bifocal. For regular seeing and walking, the person looks through the lower part of the spectacle lenses; for a magnified, clearer view of TV, faces, street signs, etc., he lowers his head slightly to look through the telescope. The usefulness of bioptics can be enhanced by adding lens "caps" which are made for looking at objects closer than three feet. It is also possible to design bioptics to see with both eyes.

Modern technology has made it possible to make the telescopes very tiny, but the principal goes back to Galileo who discovered that two lenses of opposite power, separated by a given distance, can enlarge an image. A new and interesting way to approach this is by using a contact lens combined with strong glasses, on the eye. While the possible magnification is limited, it works wonderfully for some people. The fitting of such an arrangement requires critical planning and execution. Sometimes it is combined with bioptic telescopes in the glasses for greater benefits. Dr. Solomon has done pioneering work in this field with considerable success.

GUIDE TO OPTICAL AIDS FOR THE PARTIALLY SIGHTED

Type of Aid	How Used	When Used	Comments
I. Telescopes. A. Binoculars. 1. Handheld.	One or both eyes. Adjustable focus.	For distance magnification. Distance viewing. 5 feet or more. TV, sports, faces, street signs, etc.	Available in various magnifications. Field size depends on lens size and power. Wide angle available.
	One eye only.	Near viewing. For near work and intermediate distances. Writing, reading labels on shelves, etc.	Limited to tasks of short duration. Difficult to use if hands unsteady. Small field of view.
2. Ready-made binoculars in eyeglass frame.	One or both eyes.	For distance viewing. TV, movies, theatre, sports, etc.	Available in up to 3 X magnification only. Relatively inexpensive. Can't be used if lens prescription required. Small field of view.
3. Headband type.	Fits on head. Can be worn over glasses or swung out of way.	Near viewing, 3 to 10 inches. Useful for light-sensitive eyes. Best if sight about equal in both eyes.	Fairly wide field, 2 to 4 inches, depending on power. Good stereoscopic effect. Frees use of hands.
4. Bioptics.	One or both eyes. Telescopes fused to upper part of glasses. Patient's Rx in lower.	Distance viewing as walking, driving. When normal, and magnified seeing is needed. School, travel, etc.	Up to 6 X magnification at distance. Can be worn at all times. Easy to use. Rx changes can be made. Expensive. Wide angle available. Must be accurately centered.

5. Near telescopes.	One eye only. Lens attachments for near and intermediate.	Intermediate and near viewing. Typing, music, etc.	Up to 8 X magnification. Relatively small field of view. Careful adjustment essential. Least amount of distortion.
B. Monoculars. (Handheld, attachable, fused.)	Telescopes fused to lower part of glasses and angled to permit use of both eyes. Patient's Rx in upper part.	When reading distances of 5 to 40 inches needed. Also typing, cooking, etc.	Attachable available up to 3 X magnification, fused up to 4 X, hand held up to 10 X. Inexpensive. Not for walking.
	One eye only. Can be clipped onto glasses. Adjustable focus.	Distance viewing. TV, school, sports, etc.	
II. Magnifiers. A. Monocular. 1. Clip-ons	Attached to temple or frame front. Either eye can be used. Can be flipped out of way.	Near viewing, 1½ to 40 inches. When strong near glasses needed, but bifocal not practical. Best as temporary aid when vision is changing.	Inexpensive and lightweight. Available with side shields for persons bothered by scattered light. Frees hands to hold reading material.
B. Binocular. 1. Clip-ons.	Attached to regular glasses. Available as flip-up.	Near viewing from 4 to 40 inches.	Inexpensive.
C. Spectacles.	Worn in ordinary eyeglass frame as bifocal, ½ eye or full reading glasses.	When large near field is needed. Strong powers for seeing as close as ½ inch from eye available. Two eyes can be used as close as 4 inches.	Frees hands to hold reading material. Cosmetically acceptable. Can be tinted for light sensitive persons. Not for use with small visual fields as in advanced glaucoma. Relatively inexpensive except in very strong powers.

(Available with handles, pocket size, folding type, illuminating attachments. Glass or plastic.)	distance. Can be used over bifocals. Available from 1 X to 17 X. Powers over 5 X should be held close to eyes for widest field. Can be suspended from neck to free hands.	tive about appearance of other aids. Difficult to use with unsteady hands. Holding magnifiers close to eyes enlarges field of view.
E. Stand.		
1. Fixed-focus.	Lens placed over material. Rests on a stand. Patient must use bifocal or have focusing ability.	For greater reading distances. For patient who cannot hold hand magnifier steady. Magnification from 1 X to 20 X possible. Easy to use.
2. Adjustable focus.	Must be used close to eye with attachable illumination. No bifocal needed.	When patient has very poor sight and little or no focusing ability. Very strong powers available. Very limited field of view.
III. Projection magnifiers.	Enlarges reading material by projecting it on a screen. Either optical or electronic with TV screen.	When sight is very limited. Up to 40 X magnification possible. Can be used for writing. Has typewriter attachment. Electronic magnifier is not easily portable. Very expensive. Newer devices have good quality picture with variable illumination. Can be used in comfortable sitting position.

GUIDE TO NON-OPTICAL AIDS FOR THE PARTIALLY SIGHTED

Type of Aid	How it is Used	Where Obtainable
A. Writing aids		
1. Bold lined paper	Easier to write along a straight line. Helps keep place. Available for all grades of school and for letter writing.	American Printing House for the Blind.
2. Check writing guide	For easier location of name, amount and signature on checks. Cut to order.	American Foundation for the Blind.
3. Porous tip pens	These pens write with darker, bolder lines. Easier to read your own writing. Come in many thicknesses and colors.	Most stationery, variety and department stores.
4. Letter writing guide	For proper spacing of sentences and to write in a straight line.	American Foundation for the Blind.
B. Reading, typing stands and racks		
1. Adjustable table reading stand	Convenient holder for any size book. Adjustable to many angles.	New York Association for the Blind.
2. Desk top reading stand clips	Holds any width book. Portable and can be used in classroom.	American Printing House for the Blind.
3. Adjustable reading stands	The height, angle, distance and position of reading material can be easily controlled. Also useful for music and typing.	Stationery stores.
4. Attachable reading stands.	Can be clamped to table tops, desks. Fully adjustable.	American Printing House for the Blind.

stand	material.	for the Blind.
6. Shafer reading stand.	Floor model adjustable for standing or sitting at any angle.	American Printing House for the Blind.
C. Light shields		
1. Visors	Attached to head. Protects from glare and overhead light.	Stationery, department stores.
2. Visorette	As above, but attached to glasses.	N.Y. Association for Blind.
3. Side shields	Protects from glare, dust, dirt. Fastens to sides of glasses. Opaque or tinted.	Optical houses.
4. Wrap around clip-on sunglasses	Plastic lenses clipped on the inside of frames for glare protection.	Optical houses.
5. Noir sun glasses	Only known plastic lenses which filters out infra-red rays. Two densities allow either 7% or 17% light to enter eye. Worn over glasses. Useful after cataract surgery.	Optical houses.
D. Aids for music		
1. Large type music staff paper.	For hand transcribing music.	American Printing House for the Blind.
2. Notation-draft board	Includes notes and material to construct music phrases, etc. For people with very limited sight.	American Printing House for the Blind.

GUIDE TO NON-OPTICAL AIDS FOR THE PARTIALLY SIGHTED (Continued)

3. Music racks	Designed for upright piano. Adjustable to many distances and angles.	American Printing House for the Blind
E. Large print books and publications	Wide range of material available. Fiction, non-fiction, technical, religious, etc.	Keith Jennison Books. American Printing House for the Blind. Large Print Publications, American Bible Society.
F. Dictionaries	Large print for school, home, etc.	Books, Inc. Stanwix House
G. Large print newspapers	Enlarged print New York Times published weekly.	New York Times
H. Large telephone dials	Large numbers for easier dialing.	Telephone Company, or N.Y. Association for Blind.
I. Playing cards	Standard cards with enlarged numbers.	N.Y. Association for Blind.
J. Special illumination		
1. Lamps	Adjustable gooseneck and spring arm types to concentrate light where needed.	Lamp stores, stationers.
2. High intensity lamps	Strong, small conentrated light such as Tensor, Luxo, Lightolier, etc.	Lamp stores, stationers.

Part X

SYMPTOMS AND COMPLAINTS

CHAPTER 40

LISTING OF SYMPTOMS AND COMPLAINTS

When you report a symptom or physical complaint to your doctor, it brings certain possible causes to his or her mind. They can range from minor irregularities requiring no treatment, to serious ailments requiring prompt attention. This chapter will acquaint you with the causes of many of your symptoms and complaints. With the help of the section on Common Eye Diseases And Disorders, you may be able to tentatively diagnose some, but most require professional judgment. As a word of caution—don't make the error of the beginning medical student and consider every slight symptom a sign of a fatal affliction.

Where it applies, we have clearly indicated both the common and infrequent causes of symptoms and complaints in each category.

Blurred Vision

    I. When looking at distance
        Common:
            (a) Nearsighted
            (b) Astigmatism
            (c) Farsighted (depending on amount and age)
        Infrequent:
            (a) Cataracts
            (b) Diabetes

(c) Amblyopia
(d) Drug reactions
(e) Diseases of eye or brain
(f) Congenital, hereditary abnormalities
(g) Spasm of focusing muscles

II. When looking at near
Common:
(a) Farsighted
(b) Astigmatism
(c) Presbyopia (gradual failure of focusing ability with aging)
Infrequent:
(a) Cataracts
(b) Diabetes
(c) Drug reactions
(d) Congenital, hereditary abnormalities
(e) Diseases of the eye or brain
(f) Fatigue of convergence skill

Night Blindness

The usual complaint of poor vision at night is not actually night blindness. It is a difficulty in seeing or walking around in dim light. This could be caused by:

(a) Overexposure to bright sunlight during the day
(b) A decrease in sensitivity from circulatory problems in older people
(c) Drugs (especially alcohol, tobacco)

True night blindness is a rare disease; there is a total inability to see in dim light.

Common:
(a) Vitamin A deficiency
(b) Retinal degeneration
Infrequent:
(a) Advanced glaucoma

(b) Diseases of optic nerve
(c) Psychic disorders

Distorted Vision

Objects appear to be misshaped or different in size.

Common:
  (a) Swelling or inflammation at back of eye
Infrequent:
  (a) Drug reactions (including excessive use of alcohol, tobacco)
  (b) During migraine headache attack
  (c) Retinal detachment
  (d) Neurological or brain disorders
  (e) Psychic disorders

Temporary blindness

Generally only one eye is involved. It can last from a few seconds, to hours or even days.

Common:
  (a) Blockage of blood supply to eye or brain
  (b) Psychic disorder (hysteria)

Infrequent:

  (a) Poisoning
  (b) Injury
  (c) Drug reaction (including excessive use of alcohol, tobacco)
  (d) Neurological or brain disorders

Central Vision Loss

Direct, straight ahead sight is poor, while peripheral (side) vision is retained.

Common:
- (a) Macular degeneration
- (b) Reduced blood supply or hemorrhage
- (c) Swelling or edema of macula

Infrequent:
- (a) Amblyopia
- (b) Drug reactions
- (c) Hereditary
- (d) Retinal damage as a result of excessive infrared radiation (from welding, looking at an eclipse, etc.)
- (e) Inflammation
- (f) Neurological disorders
- (g) Cysts, tumors
- (h) Retinal detachment

Side Vision Loss

Either one or both eyes can be involved. The loss may only be in a small area, the right or left half of the visual field or the entire field.

Sudden onset:
- (a) Retinal detachment
- (b) Reduced blood supply or hemorrhage
- (c) Swelling or edema

Gradual loss:
- (a) Retinal degeneration
- (b) Glaucoma
- (c) Hereditary
- (d) Injury
- (e) Neurological, brain diseases and disorders
- (f) Inflammation or disease of optic nerve

Light Flashes

Common:
(a) Hardening of the arteries or other blood

supply disturbances
          Infrequent:
             (a) Severe coughing or sneezing
             (b) May precede retinal detachment
             (c) May precede migraine or epilepsy attack
             (d) Drug reactions
             (e) Brain concussion
             (f) Irritation to retina or optic nerve
             (g) Rubbing or pressing on eyes
             (h) Inflammation or infection of retina

Double Vision

   Seeing two objects when there is really only one. The two objects may be seen next to each other, above each other or at an angle.

   I. When seen with one eye
          Common:
             (a) Lens or corneal abnormalities
          Infrequent:
             (a) Astigmatism
             (b) Torn iris
             (c) Disease or injury to cornea
             (d) Displaced lens
             (e) Early cataract changes
             (f) Psychic disorders

   II. When seen with two eyes
          Common:
             (a) Paralysis of one or more of the muscles controlling eye movements
             (b) Imbalance in action of muscles controlling eye movements
          Infrequent:
             (a) Drug reactions
             (b) Aniseikonia

  (c) Neurological and brain disorders
  (d) Following eye or brain surgery

Floating Spots

Seen as spots, threads or specks against a bright background.
  Common:
    (a) Solidified particles in vitreous, usually in older people. Quite harmless.
  Infrequent:
    (a) Inflammation
    (b) Hemorrhage in retina
    (c) May precede retinal detachment

Light Sensitivity
 I. Severe
   Common:
    (a) Foreign particle on eye
    (b) Injury to cornea
   Infrequent:
    (a) Inflammation
    (b) Drug reaction
    (c) Hereditary (such as albinism)
    (d) Enlarged pupil which doesn't constrict to light
 II. Mild
   Common:
    (a) Inflammation of lids or eye
    (b) Contact lens wear
   Infrequent:
    (a) Neuralgia, neuritis
    (b) Migraine headaches
    (c) Focusing effort fatigue
    (d) Dental problems
    (e) Extreme nearsightedness
    (f) Drug reactions or poisoning

Halos Around Lights

Rings of colors or halos around light sources. One or both eyes can be affected.
Common:
  (a) Glaucoma
  (b) Swelling of cornea (often from contact lens overwear)
  (c) Cataracts
Infrequent:
  (a) Corneal scar
  (b) Disease of cornea
  (c) Drug reactions

Pain In Eye

I. Moderate to severe

  Common:
    (a) Foreign particle on cornea or lids
    (b) Inflammation in or around the eye
  Infrequent:
    (a) Inverted eyelash
    (b) Acute glaucoma (usually with nausea)
    (c) Corneal abrasion from wearing contact lenses too long or from poor fitting contact lenses
    (d) Neuralgia (usually one side of face)
    (e) Disease or injury to cornea
    (f) Sinus infection

II. Discomfort, eye strain or dull ache
  Common:
    (a) Farsighted
    (b) Astigmatism
    (c) Presbyopia (when reading)

    (d) Imbalance of action of muscles controlling eye movements
    (e) Fatigue of focusing or eye convergence (usually in afternoon after close work)
   Infrequent:
    (a) Chronic conjunctivitis
    (b) Light glare; too much or too little light
    (c) Lack of sleep or rest
    (d) Aniseikonia
 III. Sensation of burning, itching, smarting
   Common:
    (a) Conjunctivitis
    (b) Allergies
   Infrequent:
    (a) Drug reactions
    (b) Dry eyes
    (c) Contact lens wear
    (d) Atmospheric conditions and pollutants

Headaches

 I. Associated with the use of the eyes
   Common:
    (a) Farsighted
    (b) Astigmatism
    (c) Imbalance of action of muscles controlling eye movements
    (d) Fatigue of focusing or eye convergence (usually after prolonged close work)
   Infrequent:
    (a) Aniseikonia
 II. Not associated with use of the eyes
   Common:
    (a) Neuralgia (usually one side of head)
    (b) Sinus infection
    (c) High or low blood pressure

(d) General fatigue
(e) Too much alcohol, overeating, etc.
(f) General disease or infection
(g) Migraine (one side of head)

Redness

I. Lids

> Common:
> (a) Styes
> (b) Allergies
> (c) Conjunctivitis
>
> Infrequent:
> (a) Insect bite
> (b) Blocked tear duct
> (c) Inflammation of any of the numerous lid glands

II. Eye

> Common:
> (a) Hemorrhage of small blood vessel from injury or disease (shows up dramatically against white of eye)
> (b) Inflammation or disease
> (c) Acute conjunctivitis
>
> Infrequent:
> (a) Acute glaucoma

Secretions and Discharges

I. Excessive tearing

> Common:
> (a) Irritation to cornea
> (b) Allergies

(c) Wind or cold weather
(d) Blocked tear drainage system
(e) In older people, loose lower lid
(f) Psychic

Infrequent:
(a) Inflammation
(b) Bright light or glare
(c) Chemical irritants
(d) Poorly fitting contact lenses
(e) Disease of tear gland
(f) Imbalance of muscles controlling eye movements
(g) Reading strain

II. Unusual discharges (pus, mucous, etc.)

Common:
(a) Conjunctivitis
(b) Allergies
(c) Inflammation of lid margin

Infrequent:
(a) Dry eyes
(b) Infections
(c) Inflammation of lid glands
(d) Chemical irritants

Frequent Blinking

Common:
(a) Together with a facial tic, a habit in some children

Infrequent:
(a) Older people with dry eyes
(b) Nervous system disease

Change In Pupil Size

I. Dilated (large)

Common:
- (a) In dim light
- (b) Drug reactions
- (c) Disease or injury to nervous system
- (d) Psychological (pleasure, fear, etc.)

Infrequent:
- (a) Glaucoma
- (b) Tumors of brain
- (c) Coma as from diabetes, epilepsy, etc.
- (d) Diseases of the retina

II. Constricted (small)

Common:
- (a) In bright light
- (b) Normal condition in older people
- (c) Drug reactions (including too much alcohol)

Infrequent:
- (a) General diseases such as syphilis, diabetes, multiple sclerosis
- (b) Diseases of central nervous system
- (c) Psychological

Small Lumps

I. Lids

Common:
- (a) Sty (Swelling near lid margin growing into small lump. Comes to a yellowish head, breaks open and discharges matter. Heals quickly
- (b) Cysts

Infrequent:
- (a) Tumors and fatty tissue accumulation

II. Eye
    Common:
        (a) Cysts
        (b) Fatty deposits
    Infrequent:
        (a) Tumors

Colored Spots On White Of Eye

    Common:
        (a) Pigmented tumors
        (b) Small blood vessel loops
        (c) Pinguecula
        (d) Small hemorrhage
    Infrequent:
        (a) Inflammation
        (b) Vitamin A deficiency
        (c) Drug reactions
        (d) Thinned areas of white cover tissue
        (e) After surgery

Eyelids

    I. Droopy. Generally only one lid is affected.
        Common:
            (a) Hereditary
            (b) With aging, loss of muscle tone and decrease of fatty tissue.
        Infrequent:
            (a) Paralyzed lid muscle
            (b) Neurological disorder
            (c) General diseases
            (d) Tumors
            (e) Hemorrhage
            (f) Insect bite (temporary swelling may give appearance of droop)
            (g) After lid or eye surgery

II. Swelling
- Common:
    - (a) Allergies
    - (b) Inflammation
    - (c) Problems with blood supply
- Infrequent:
    - (a) Insect bite
    - (b) Infections
    - (c) Reactions to vaccines, penicillin, etc.
    - (d) Swollen tear gland
    - (e) Tumors
    - (f) Injury

III. Baggy (loose folds of skin)
- (a) Hereditary
- (b) Weight loss

IV. Margins turn inward or outward
- (a) Congenital
- (b) Allergies
- (c) Aging process
- (d) Scar tissue
- (e) Spasm of lid muscles

Protruding Eyeball

I. When both eyes are involved
- Common:
    - (a) Overactive thyroid

II. When one eye is involved
- (a) Swelling
- (b) Inflammation
- (c) Tumors
- (d) Injury

Shrinking Eyeball

Generally, the eyeball is not getting smaller, but only gives that appearance because the fatty tissue around the globe is diminishing.

    (a) In aged persons
    (b) Following cataract surgery
    (c) Injury

A true sunken eyeball is blind.

    (a) Congenital
    (b) Disease
    (c) Injury
    (d) Tumors

Eye Oscillations

The rapid movements may be back and forth, up and down, or mixed.

    Common:
        (a) Congenital
    Infrequent:
        (a) Diseases of the brain and nervous system
        (b) Tumors of the brain and nervous system

GLOSSARY

Abberation: The failure of refracted light to focus to a common point.
Abrasion: An erosion of the surface cell layers. (See corneal abrasion.)
Accommodation: The "automatic" adjustment the eye makes in order to focus on objects at different distances.
After-image: An image which remains after the light stimulation to the retina has stopped. It is called positive when seen as the original, negative when dark and light are reversed or colors are seen as complimentary.
Amaurosis: Blindness caused by any disease.
Amblyopia: Poor sight in a healthy eye which does not fully improve with a corrective spectacle or contact lens. The most common type, ex-anopsia, is due to lack of use/suppression. It can also be toxic, caused by poisons.
Ametropia: Any sight problem caused by an improperly focused image on the retina.
Aniridia: A congenital lack of the iris.
Aniseikonia: The images seen by each eye are different in size or shape.
Anisocoria: The pupils are of unequal size.
Anisometropia: The two eyes have an unequal refractive power.
Anomalous fixation: An eye which uses an area other than the fovea for sighting.
Anterior chamber: Fluid-filled space between the cornea and the lens of the eye.
Antimetropia: One eye is farsighted, the other nearsighted.
Aphakia: The lens of the eye is lacking.
Aqueous humor: A clear, watery fluid filling the anterior chamber. It carries nutrients to the lens and cornea, and removes waste material.
Arcus senilis: A whitish circle or arc at the border of the cornea. Very common in the aging, but harmless.
Arteriosclerosis: Hardening of the arteries.
Asthenopia: A catch-all term to describe discomfort associated with fatigue of the visual system.

Astigmatism:	A refractive condition which causes parts of an object to focus at different distances behind the lens of the eye. Therefore, the entire object cannot be in focus at the same time. Usually it's caused by an "out of round" cornea.
Atrophy:	The wasting away of cells or tissues from lack of nutrition.
Atropine:	A drug used to temporarily dilate the pupil and paralyze accommodation.
Bifocal:	A spectacle or contact lens with two focusing distances—one for far, one for near.
Binocular vision:	The ability of the brain to fuse the images from each eye into a single percept.
Biomicroscope:	An instrument for examining the front and interior of the eye under magnification.
Blepharitis:	An inflammation of the eyelids.
Blepharospasm:	A twitching of the eyelids, often due to eye strain.
Blind spot:	The natural blind area of the retina where the optic nerve enters the eye.
Campimeter:	An instrument for determining the integrity of the central field of vision.
Canthus:	The junction of the eyelids.
Cataract:	An opaqueness in the lens of the eye.
Chalazion:	A small cyst or enlargement of a lid gland.
Choroid:	The middle-layer tissue of the eyeball.
Chromatic abberation:	A dispersion of light into its component colors.
Ciliary body:	Part of the inner layer of the eye to which the lens is attached. Contraction of the ciliary muscle permits the lens to accommodate.
Color deficiency:	The inability to correctly identify all colors.
Cone:	The light sensitive cell of the retina, mostly in the central macula region which responds to colors.
Conjunctiva:	The mucous membrane lining the "white" of the eye and the inside of the lids.
Conjunctivitis:	An inflammation of the conjunctiva.
Convergence:	The act of rotating both eyes inward to look at a nearby object.
Contact lens:	A lens which fits directly on the front of the eye.
Cornea:	The transparent front portion of the eye.
Corneal abrasion:	An erosion of the front surface of the cornea, frequently causing pain and tearing.

Crystalline lens:	The transparent, elastic lens within the eye, situated immediately behind the iris.
Cycloplegia:	A paralysis of the ciliary muscles. Suspends accommodation and dilates the pupil.
Cyclitis:	An inflammation of the ciliary body.
Cylinder lens:	A lens ground to give no power along one axis and maximum power at right angles to that axis.
Dacryoadenitis:	An inflammation of the lacrimal gland.
Dacryocystitis:	An inflammation of the lacrimal sac.
Depth perception:	The quality of seeing objects as three-dimensional solids in space. True depth perception requires the brain to fuse the images from both eyes.
Diopter:	The unit of measure for the power of a lens to bend light. A +1.00 lens will focus light to a point one meter away.
Diplopia:	Double vision.
Divergence:	Outward rotation of the eyes away from each other.
Duction:	The reserve ability of the eyes to turn inward or outward and still maintain single, binocular vision.
Dyslexia:	Difficulty in reading due to a brain disorder.
Ectropion:	Outward eversion of the lid margin.
Edema:	A tissue swelling from fluid accumulation.
Embolism:	A blood vessel blocked by a clot.
Emmetropia:	Light comes to a perfect focus on the retina with accommodation at rest.
Enophthalmos:	A deep seated or sunken eyeball.
Entropion:	Inward eversion of the lid margin.
Error of refraction:	Light from a distant object does not come to a perfect focus on the retina when the eye is in a relaxed or unaccommodated state.
Esophoria:	A tendency for the eyes to turn inward towards each other.
Esotropia:	A crossed eye condition with one eye deviating inward.
Exophoria:	A tendency for the eyes to turn outward away from each other.
Exotropia:	A crossed eye condition with one eye deviating outward. Also known as "wall-eyed."
Exophthalmos:	A protrusion or bulging of the eyeball.
Extrinsic muscles:	The six muscles attached to the outside globe of the eye which control all eye movements.

Field of vision: The total area of space seen by one eye (monocular) or by both eyes (binocular).
Fixation: The act of directing the visual gaze at an object in space.
Floaters: Small, solidified particles in the vitreous, which can be seen as spots or threads against any bright background.
Fluorescin: A harmless dye which glows green in ultraviolet light. Used to evaluate fit of contact lenses, condition of cornea and retinal blood supply.
Focal point: The point at which distant light comes to a focus after being reflected or refracted.
Focal length: The distance between a lens or mirror and its focal point.
Fovea: A tiny depression in the center of the macula region of the retina. This is the area of keenest sight.
Fundus: The inside back of the eye visible with an ophthalmoscope.
Fusion: The conversion by the brain of the images from the two eyes into one image.
Glare: Concentrated light, much brighter than the surrounding illumination.
Glaucoma: A disease caused by an increased fluid pressure within the eye, resulting in field of vision loss.
Gonioscopy: A method of examining the angle between the cornea and iris in the anterior chamber.
Hemianopsia: Blindness in one half of the visual field.
Heterochromia: The left and right eyes each have a different color iris.
Heterophoria: A tendency for one or both eyes to deviate or cross.
Heterotropia: A condition wherein the eyes do not "point" together.
Hordeolum (sty): Infection of a lash follicle of the lid margin.
Horopter: The field of vision seen binocularly in three-dimension when fixating at a given point.
Hyperemia: Congestion of the blood vessels from an infection, inflammation or surgery.
Hypermetropia, hyperopia: Farsighted. An eye whose refractive power is too weak for its length.
Hyperphoria: A tendency for an eye to deviate upward.
Hypertensive retinopathy: A vascular disease of the retina associated with general high bood pressure.

Hypertropia:	One eye is deviated upward.
Hypophoria:	A tendency for one eye to deviate downward.
Hypopion:	An accumulation of pus at the bottom of the anterior chamber.
Hypotropia:	One eye is deviated downward.
Infra-red:	Invisible electro-magnetic radiation with a wavelength just beyond visible red light. Can be felt as heat.
Intraocular tension:	The pressure of the fluid within the eye.
Iridectomy:	Surgical removal of a part of the iris.
Iris:	The thin, colored circular membrane of the eye, located in front of the lens. Its central black opening is the pupil.
Iritis:	Inflammation of the iris.
Keratitis:	Inflammation of the cornea.
Keratoconous:	Thinning of the cornea near the center, resulting in a cone-shaped bulge.
Keratometer:	An instrument for measuring the central area curvature of the cornea. Same as ophthalmometer.
Kryptok:	The name of one of the earliest types of fused bifocal lenses.
Lacrimal apparatus:	The tear-producing and disposal system of the eye.
Lagophthalmos:	An inability to fully close the lids.
Lamina cribrosa:	A perforated area of the choroid layer through which the optic nerve enters the eye.
Lens:	(a) An optical device to transmit or bend light. (b) The small, transparent, circular, elastic body in the eye involved with focusing.
Leucoma:	A whitish opacity of the cornea.
Luxation:	A condition where the lens of the eye is displaced from its normal position.
Macropsia:	A condition where objects are seen larger than they really are.
Macula:	The most sensitive retinal area for sight and color vision.
Macular degeneration:	Partial or total loss of this sensitive retinal area (macula) resulting in reduced sight. Most common in the aged.
Micropsia:	A condition where objects are seen smaller than they really are.
Miosis:	A condition where the pupil becomes smaller.

Monocular:	Having only one eye.
Monocular vision:	Seeing with only one eye.
Muscae volitantes:	Floating spots seen against any bright background.
Multifocal:	A spectacle or contact lens with more than one focusing power area.
Mydriasis:	A condition where the pupil becomes larger.
Mydriatic:	A drug used to dilate the pupil.
Myopia:	Nearsighted. An eye whose refractive power is too strong for its length.
Near point:	The closest point which the eye is capable of accommodating. This point gradually recedes with age.
Night blindness:	An inability to see at night or in dim illumination.
Nystagmus:	Involuntary oscillation of the eye.
Oculist:	A physician who specializes in disorders and diseases of the eyes.
O.D.:	(a) Abbreviation for Latin *oculus dexter*, the right eye. (b) Following a name, the degree, Doctor of Optometry.
Opacity:	Lack of transparency resulting in blockage of light. Usually refers to changes in the lens of the eye leading to cataracts.
Ophthalmologist:	A medical specialist dealing primarily with diseases and surgery of the eyes.
Ophthalmometer:	An instrument for measuring the central area curvature of the cornea. Same as keratometer.
Ophthalmoplegia:	Widespread paralysis of the eye muscles.
Ophthalmoscope:	An instrument used to inspect the inside of the eye.
Optic atrophy:	Degeneration of the optic nerve fibers with partial or complete sight loss.
Optic disc:	The area of the retina where the optic nerve and blood supply enters the eye.
Optic nerve:	The collection of about one million nerve fibers connecting each eye to the brain.
Optician:	A person who grinds lenses and deals in optical goods.
Optometrist:	A specialist skilled in the detection of eye diseases; in the diagnosis and treatment of disorders of the eyes and visual system.
Orbit:	The bony socket which surrounds the eye.

Orthophoria:	Straight eyes without any tendency for either eye to deviate.
Orthoptics:	Scientifically planned eye exercises to straighten the eyes and develop binocularity.
O.S.:	Abbreviation for Latin *oculus sinister*, left eye.
O.U.:	Abbreviation for Latin *oculus uterque*, both eyes.
Papillitis:	An inflammation of the optic disc.
Paresis:	A slight or partial paralysis.
Perimetry:	The measurement of the extent and integrity of the visual field.
Peripheral vision:	The ability to perceive objects and movements away from the direct line of sight.
Photophobia:	An intolerance to light.
Photopsia:	Seeing flashing lights which are not physically present.
Pinguecula:	A small, yellowish elevation on the conjunctiva.
Pink eye:	A common term for an acute conjunctivitis.
Pleoptics:	Light stimulation therapy in the treatment of amblyopia.
Presbyopia:	Decreased ability of the eye, with age, to focus near objects and printed material.
Prism:	A lens which displaces or bends light in one direction.
Pterygium:	A triangular shaped, vascular growth on the conjunctiva near the limbus, which may overgrow the cornea.
Ptosis:	A drooping of the upper lid.
Pupil:	The small, black circular opening in the iris through which light enters the eye.
Refraction:	The bending of light as it passes from a medium of one density to that of another.
Refractive error:	A defect in the refractive system of the eye which prevents light from coming to a clear, sharp focus on the retina.
Retina:	The inner layer of the eye containing the light sensitive cells and numerous nerve cells.
Retinoscope:	An instrument used to measure the refractive power of the eye objectively.
Retrobulbar neuritis:	An inflammation of the optic nerve behind the optic disc.
Rods:	The light sensitive cells of the retina which respond to light, dark, movements, shapes, but not to colors.

Sclera:	The outer white covering of the eye.
Scotoma:	A blind or partially missing area in the visual field.
Snellen chart:	A letter or number chart for scientifically measuring the central visual acuity.
Slit lamp:	See biomicroscope.
Squint:	(a) To look with the eyes partially closed. (b) A deviating eye.
Stereopsis:	Seeing objects in three dimension. The end result of the brain fusing the images from both eyes.
Strabismus:	The two eyes are not "pointing" together. Concomitant, when the eyes move together even though one is deviated; non-concomitant (paralytic), when the deviating eye does not move together with the pointing eye.
Sty:	The common name for hordeolum.
Subluxation:	Partially displaced lens of the eye.
Synechia:	Adhesion of the iris to the lens or cornea.
Tachistoscope:	An instrument used in visual therapy to enlarge the span of visual recognition.
Tangent screen:	An instrument used to examine the central visual field for scotomas and other abnormalities.
Temple:	The arm or handle of an eyeglass frame which fits over the ear.
Thrombosis:	Blood clot obstruction in a vessel.
Tonometer:	An instrument for measuring the fluid pressure within the eye.
Trachoma:	A viral disease of the conjunctival lining of the lids resulting in a cobblestone appearance and causing scarring of the cornea.
Trichiasis:	A condition in which the eyelashes grow inward towards the cornea.
Trifocal:	A lens with three distinct focusing areas.
Tropia:	A deviated or crossed eye.
Uvea:	The choroid, ciliary body and iris of the eye.
Uveitis:	An inflammation of the uvea.
Ultra-violet:	Highly energetic, invisible electro-magnetic radiation with a wavelength adjacent to visible violet. Responsible for skin tanning; can cause eye damage.
Visual acuity:	The sharpness of sight, usually measured in the Snellen fractions 20/20, 20/80, etc.

Visual axis:	Direction of gaze.
Visual illusion:	Misinterpretation by the brain of a visual setting or scene.
Vitreous humor:	A transparent, jelly-like substance which fills the eye behind the lens.
Vertical phoria:	The tendency for an eye to deviate upward or downward.
Visual Therapy:	Various types of scientific training procedures geared to improve the functioning of the visual system.
Wall eyed:	One eye deviates outward.
Xanthelasma:	A flat, yellowish growth on the lids.
Xerosis:	Abnormal dryness of the eye.
Zonule of Zinn:	Thin, threadlike ligaments which hold the lens in place within the eye.

MAR 1978

NO LONGER PROPERTY OF
CAMBRIA COUNTY LIBRARY